W9-CFP-830

praise for the first edition of
How to Be Sick

"This is a book for all of us."

—SYLVIA BOORSTEIN,

author of *Happiness Is an Inside Job*

"An immensely wise book. Health psychology has been poisoned by the view that the best way to approach illness is through a muscular, militant resistance. Toni Bernhard reveals how letting go, surrendering, and putting the ego aside yield insights and fulfillment even in the presence of illness. A major contribution."

—LARRY DOSSEY, MD,

author of *Healing Words*

"A profound, compassionate, and intimate guide for living wisely."

—GIL FRONSDAL,

author of *The Issue at Hand*

"When we lose our physical health, it can seem like we've lost our life. Toni Bernhard, with unflinching realness and deep insight, shows us how the fires of loss can clear the way for a new and profound capacity for appreciation, love, and understanding. This book can bring you more fully alive by healing your spirit."

—TARA BRACH,

author of *Radical Acceptance*

"Told with relentless honesty and clarity."

—STEPHEN BATCHELOR,

author of *Buddhism Without Beliefs*

"An encouraging book that treats sickness as something to welcome because, when you are sick, that is the obstacle that has to be your gate. This book is full of compassion about how to sit sweetly with your difficulties—which means not making yourself wrong for *having* difficulties."

—JOHN TARRANT,
author of *The Light Inside the Dark*

"Toni Bernhard offers a lifeline to those whose lives have been devastated by illness, and shows us all how to transform suffering into peace and even joy."

—LYNN ROYSTER FUENTES,
founder of the Chronic Illness Initiative at DePaul University

"A road map to finding grace and balance amid affliction."

—CHRISTINA FELDMAN,
author of *Boundless Heart*

"Practical, wise, and full of heart."

—JAMES BARAZ,
author of *Awakening Joy*

"This warm and engaging book can help with even the most difficult situation."

—THOMAS BIEN, PHD,
author of *Mindful Recovery*

"*How to Be Sick* is a good friend to keep close by so that illness doesn't become the enemy."

—ED & DEB SHAPIRO,
authors of *The Unexpected Power of Mindfulness and Meditation*

"Don't pass up this book—and don't be misled by the title. This book isn't about being sick as much as it as about living right now. This practical yet exceedingly graceful book is a love story—about life, the endurance of the human spirit, and the power of a sustaining relationship."

—ALIDA BRILL,
author of *Dancing at the River's Edge*

"Living a life of peace and contentment is not difficult when life is cooperating—but what happens when the reality of our lives is suddenly turned upside down and shaken by hardship or affliction? This book is an inspiring and instructive guide for coping with a chronic condition or life-threatening illness, but it is much more than that. Each chapter is about unpacking the highest truth in the lowest places of our lives.
The book is called *How to Be Sick*, but it's really about how to live."

—JIM PALMER,
author of *Divine Nobodies*

"An intimate, gripping, profound, and eminently useful book about being joyfully and wisely alive no matter what happens to you."

—RICK HANSON, PHD,
author of *Buddha's Brain*

"Who would have thought that there is a 'how to' for being sick? But now there is! Deeply moving and impressive. I highly recommend her book as a must-read for anyone who is ill or caring for someone ill. Her gifts will transform you."

—LEWIS RICHMOND,
author of *Aging as a Spiritual Practice*

"A warm and compassionate guide for navigating illness on a personal and practical level, a level physicians rarely see or discuss with their patients. The greatest compliment I could give this book is that I will be recommending it to all of my chronically ill patients as a guide for remaining happy even in the absence of good health."

—ALEX LICKERMAN, MD,
former director of primary care at the University of Chicago

"A unique and creative adaptation of spiritual practice to the challenges of chronic illness. *How to Be Sick* is a wise, compassionate book that will help all of us live well."

—DOROTHY WALL,
author of *Encounters with the Invisible*

"Each of us finds our way to live with the challenges and uncertainty of illness. Toni Bernhard found a path that led to balance, wisdom, and love. She caringly points us to the possibility of finding happiness even in the midst of difficult conditions. That is a true gift."

—FRANK OSTASESKI,
founder of the Metta Institute

"An eloquent and compelling account. This book is a major achievement."

—*Spirituality and Practice*

"Very compelling—great teaching interwoven into the heartful human drama of family, illness, and day-to-day life."

—SHAILA CATHERINE,
author of *Focused and Fearless*

"A must-read with a solid dose of hope."
—LORI HARTWELL,
author of *Chronically Happy*

"Everyone should read this book—anyone who is sick, anyone who loves someone who is sick, and anyone who has ever experienced things being other than they'd hoped they would be. Toni Bernhard openheartedly shares the deep pain and equally deep joy of her experience in a way that allows us to validate the pain of our own circumstances, and still find joy and contentment within any context.

"She offers simple, deeply wise practices that reduce the suffering associated with grasping for things to be other than they are by allowing us to accept and enjoy things exactly as they are, including our own desire for something else. Her willingness to step fully into her life after it's been dramatically narrowed by illness, and to share this process with us, inspires us each to live our own lives more fully, accepting the challenges that arise, and finding the joys inherent in each moment.

"I plan to buy a copy for everyone I love."
—LIZABETH ROEMER, PHD,
coauthor of *The Mindful Way through Anxiety*

"Readers need not be Buddhist or meditators to benefit from Toni's wisdom."
—Cheri Register,
author of *The Chronic Illness Experience*

"You don't have to be sick to benefit from the advice in this book. This is a book on how to live fully."
—JOY SELAK, author of *You Don't LOOK Sick!*

How to Be Sick

How to Be Sick

A Buddhist-Inspired Guide
for the Chronically Ill
and Their Caregivers

REVISED AND UPDATED EDITION

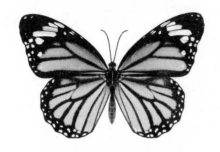

Toni Bernhard

Foreword by Sylvia Boorstein

Wisdom Publications
199 Elm Street
Somerville MA 02144 USA
www.wisdompubs.org

© 2018 Toni Bernhard

All rights reserved.

No part of this book may be reproduced in any form or by any means, electronic or mechanical, including photography, recording, or by any information storage and retrieval system or technologies now known or later developed, without permission in writing from the publisher.

The Library of Congress has cataloged the earlier edition as follows:
Bernhard, Toni.
 How to be sick : a Buddhist-inspired guide for the chronically ill and their caregivers / Toni Bernhard.
    p. cm.
Includes bibliographical references and index.
ISBN 0-86171-626-4 (pbk. : alk. paper)
 1. Religious life—Buddhism. 2. Chronically ill—Religious life. 3. Caregivers—Religious life. 4. Chronic diseases—Religious aspects—Buddhism. I. Title.
BQ5400.B46 2010
294.3'4442—dc22

                        2010025648

21 20 19 18   5 4 3 2 1

ISBN 978-1-61429-478-8   eBook ISBN 978-1-61429-503-7

Cover design by Philip Pascuzzo.
Interior design by Gopa & Ted 2, Inc. Set in Sabon LT Std 11/16.

"To Know the Dark" copyright © 1985 by Wendell Berry from *The Collected Poems of Wendell Berry*, 1957–1982. Reprinted by permission of Counterpoint. Author photo by TJ.

Wisdom Publications' books are printed on acid-free paper and meet the guidelines for permanence and durability of the Production Guidelines for Book Longevity of the Council on Library Resources.

♻ This book was produced with environmental mindfulness. For more information, please visit our website, www.wisdompubs.org.

Printed in the United States of America.

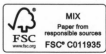

Please visit www.fscus.org.

For Tony

In sickness and in health,
to love and to cherish,
till death do us part.

Contents

Foreword

"YOU ARE GOING TO BE OKAY!" Words of reassurance are the first therapy offered to people who awaken after a surgery, or are revived after an accident, or just before the disclosure of a fearful diagnosis. "You are going to be okay" often goes along with the summary of what now needs to happen to make things better. "You'll need to stay a few more days in the hospital and then you can go home and finish recuperating there." Or, "We're on the way to the hospital and the doctors there are ready for you." Or, "We'll do chemo and then radiation and it might be a hard year but the chances are good that you'll be your old self again afterward." "You are going to be okay," in these circumstances, means "Things are uncomfortable now, but you will get well. You will be better." But it doesn't always happen that way.

This is a book for people who will not be their old self again and for all those for whom, at least now, getting better *isn't* possible. This is a book that most reassuringly says even to those people, "You, too, are going to be okay—even if you never recover your health!"

Toni Bernhard is the perfect person to write this book. In the middle of a vibrant, complex, gratifying family and professional life—literally from one day to the next—she took ill with a hard-to-diagnose and basically incurable, painfully fatiguing illness that waxes and wanes in its intensity, that sometimes seems to respond to a new treatment and then doesn't after all, that doesn't get worse but also never gets better. Years after the onset of her illness, she is still sick. She knows the cycle of hoping and feeling disappointed from the inside out as well as the cycles of deciding to give up hope in order to avoid the pain of disappointment and the sadness, and then the relief, of surrender.

Decades ago, a friend of mine, a man with a family and friends and flourishing career, said of his unexpected, debilitating illness, "This isn't what I wanted—but it's what I got." He said it matter-of-factly, without bitterness, as if he understood that it was the only reasonable response. I knew that he was telling me something important. It is a fundamental human truth, transcending cultures and traditions, that the wisest response to situations that are beyond our control, circumstances that we cannot change, is noncontention. In this book, Toni shows how her longtime study and meditation practice in the Buddhist tradition help her accommodate her situation with gentle acceptance and compassion. The techniques that Toni presents for working with one's mind in the distressed states it finds itself when facing an uncomfortable and unchangeable truth are basic Buddhist insights and meditation practices, but they are nonparochial. They will work for anyone.

This book is written for people who are ill and aren't going to get better, and also for their caregivers, people who love them and suffer along with them in wishing that things were different. It speaks most specifically about physical illness. In the largest sense, though, I feel that this book is for all of us. Sooner or later, we all are going to not "get better." Speaking as an older person who has had the good fortune of health, I know that the core challenge in my life, and, I believe, in all of our lives, from beginning to end,

xvi   How to Be Sick

is accommodating to realities that we wish were other, and doing it with grace.

Toni has given us a gift by sharing her life and her wisdom, and I am grateful for it.

Sylvia Boorstein

Preface to the Revised Edition

I T'S BEEN EIGHT YEARS since *How to Be Sick* was published. I had no idea that what began as a collection of notes to myself about how to make the best of living with chronic illness would turn into a book with a worldwide following.

I undertook the work involved in preparing a new edition for two principal reasons: to clarify the ideas and practices from the original book and to share new ones. To that end, every chapter has either been rewritten, expanded, or revised. There's a lot of new material in this book!

In addition, when *How to Be Sick* was first published, I assumed its audience would be mostly Buddhist. To my surprise and delight, this has not turned out to be the case. People from all (or no) spiritual and religious persuasions have been helped by my Buddhist-inspired approach and the practices I offer. Because I underestimated the audience, the first edition was full of "Buddhist" words from two languages—Pali, the written form of the Buddha's language, and Sanskrit. People ask me in emails, "What was that word you used for 'compassion' again?" Well, in this edition, when a Pali word translates clearly and adequately into

English, I use the English word. And so, the word for "compassion" is now . . . compassion!

Finally, I wrote *How to Be Sick* with only physical pain and illness in mind. Yet many people have written to me about how the book has helped them or a loved one cope with chronic mental illness, such as anxiety, depression, bipolar disorder, or PTSD. I want to be sure they feel included in this new edition.

In the past eight years, some of my health issues have remained the same. I still have the chronic illness that you'll read about in the first two "autobiographical" chapters of the book. But I've also been coping with some new health problems that have increased my pain levels, sometimes dramatically.

The major health event for me since the first edition was published is that I was diagnosed with breast cancer in November 2014. I underwent a lumpectomy and a course of radiation treatment. My prognosis is good, but the episode has worsened my longtime illness, and I also struggle to cope with the side effects of the medication I take to prevent a recurrence. I've learned that breast cancer, too, is a chronic illness.

After the first two chapters, I limit discussing my personal health to places in the text where I think my experience will help you, the reader, understand a point I'm making or a practice I'm describing. *How to Be Sick* was never intended to be a memoir. It's a practical guide. In this new edition, I've continued to try to strike a balance between personal stories and keeping the text focused on chronic illness in general.

My readers struggle with a vast array of mental and physical problems. Despite this, I've learned in the past eight years that we have more in common than we have differences. No matter where we live in the world, no matter what educational level we've reached, no matter what our financial situation is, no matter how much support we get from family and friends, we're in this together.

It warms my heart and lifts my spirits to be able to help people with my writing. Some days, that's what keeps me going. My deep thanks to each and every one of you.

Toni Bernhard

Preface to the First Edition

One, seven, three, five—
Nothing to rely on in this or any world;
Nighttime falls and the water is flooded with moonlight.
Here in the Dragon's jaws:
Many exquisite jewels.
—SETCHO JUKEN

IN MAY OF 2001, I got sick and never recovered.

The summer of 2008 marked my seventh year of living with chronic illness. One night that summer, at about ten P.M., my husband came into our bedroom and joined me on the bed that has become my home. My husband's parents named him Tony; my parents named me Toni. We met when we were dating each other's roommates in college. On the morning of November 22, 1963, he knocked on my apartment door with the news that President Kennedy had been assassinated. Tony and I have been inseparable ever since. By ten P.M., I'm in what we call "stun-gun" state—as if I've been hit with a Taser—meaning it's often hard for me to move my body and do anything other than stare blankly into space.

I greeted him with, "I wish I weren't sick."

Tony replied, "I wish you weren't sick."

There was a slight pause, then we both started laughing.

"Okay. That got said."

It was a breakthrough moment for the two of us.

We'd had this exchange dozens of times since the summer of 2001, but it took seven long years for the exchange to bring us to laughter instead of to sorrow and, often, to tears. This book is intended to help the chronically ill and their caregivers move from tears to laughter. Not always laughter, of course, but laughter enough. (Please note that in my writing, "chronic illness" includes chronic pain.) The book's coverage includes the following:

- ▸ weathering the relentlessness of symptoms
- ▸ coming to terms with a more isolated life
- ▸ coping with emotional distress, especially fear about the future
- ▸ handling the misunderstanding of others
- ▸ dealing with the health-care system; and
- ▸ for spouses, partners, or other caregivers, adapting to so many unexpected and sometimes sudden life changes.

In chapters 1 and 2, I write about how I got sick and, to Tony's and my own bewilderment, stayed sick. Starting in chapter 3, I describe how, drawing on the teachings of the Buddha, I learned the spiritual practice of "how to be sick," meaning how to live a life of purpose and joy despite my physical and energetic limitations. I offer simple practices, ranging from those that are traditionally Buddhist to others I devised after becoming chronically ill. I also include a chapter on Byron Katie's work, which I have found particularly helpful.

You need not be a Buddhist to benefit from the practices in this book. If a suggested practice resonates with you, truly "practice" it. Work with it over and over until it enters your heart, mind, and body and becomes a natural response to the difficulties you face as the result of being chronically ill or being the caregiver of a chronically ill person.

At the end of the book, I've provided a quick reference guide that matches specific challenges faced by the chronically ill and their caregivers to practices described in the book.

I put this book together slowly and with great difficulty. I wrote it lying on my bed, laptop on my stomach, notes strewn about on the blanket, printer within arm's reach. Some days, I would get so involved in a chapter that I'd work too long. The result would be an exacerbation of my symptoms that would leave me unable to write at all for several days or even for weeks.

There were also periods when I was simply too sick or in pain to even think of putting a book together. Then the project would be left untouched for months on end. Feeling so unwell physically would sometimes have such a strong effect on me mentally that, during the darkest moments, I considered tossing out all the work I'd done, despairing of ever being able to complete it.

But painful thoughts and emotions come and go. In the end, I pressed on, determined to finish the book in the hope it would help others. The Buddha's teachings have inspired and comforted me for many years. The Buddha and the schools that his teachings gave rise to offer many simple yet powerful practices that guide both the healthy and the chronically ill through life's ups and downs.

The inspiration to write this book came from a person I knew for such a short time and in such limited circumstances that I don't even know how to spell her name. In 1999, I was on a ten-day silent meditation retreat at Spirit Rock Meditation Center.

As always on retreat, each of us had what's called "work meditation," meaning we are responsible for performing a task each day to help the retreat run smoothly. Some people cut vegetables, some wash dishes, others clean the bathrooms. As much as possible, we maintain silence even if we work alongside others.

My work meditation was to clear the trays from the serving tables in the dining hall after lunch and put the leftovers in containers. I shared this job with a woman who introduced herself as Marianne and was about my age. She looked a bit frail to me, but we shared the work equally, only speaking in a whisper now and then: "Is this container big enough to hold the extra salad?" In the meditation hall, I noticed that she seemed to be with a young man who might be her son. I remember thinking how nice it was that they were here together. She had a kind face and a gentle smile and I looked forward to seeing her every day after lunch.

In addition to working in the dining hall, we followed a path to a small building where the teachers ate and then we brought their serving trays back to the kitchen. On the seventh day of the retreat, to my surprise, another woman accompanied Marianne. The three of us cleared the serving tables in the dining hall and then the new woman followed me outside as I began to walk down to the teachers' dining room. She asked, "Do you know about Marianne?"

When I shook my head, she told me, "She's very sick. She only has a couple of weeks to live." Then she turned around and went back into the dining hall. I continued to the teachers' dining room, shaken by this unexpected discovery. There, on the path, was one of the teachers. In my distress, I broke the silence. I asked her if she knew about Marianne. She replied that Marianne was here with her son. Then she told me something she probably shouldn't have (which is why I'm not using her name). She said that on the information sheet we fill out when we get to the retreat, under the question that asks if there's anything the teachers should know about us, Marianne had written, "I have just two weeks to live but it won't affect my practice."

The next day Marianne's spot and her son's spot in the meditation hall were empty.

In memory of Marianne, I vow to do my best not to let my illness affect my practice. I also vow to let my practice continue to teach me how to be sick—and to enable me to help others who are chronically ill as well as those who care for them.

Toni Bernhard

How Everything Changed

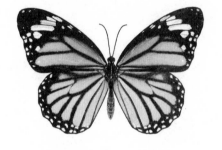

I

Getting Sick

A ROMANTIC TRIP TO PARIS

Paris ain't much of a town.

—BABE RUTH

At the end of August 2001, I was to begin my twentieth year as a law professor at the University of California at Davis. To celebrate and to treat ourselves, Tony and I decided to go on a special vacation. Surfing the Internet, I found a studio apartment in Paris for rent at a reasonable price. We were not world travelers: a trip to Paris was a big deal for us. For three weeks, we'd immerse ourselves in the life and culture of the City of Lights. We were going to have a great time.

At the airport things got off to an inauspicious start. As we sat in our seats on the United Airlines commuter flight from Sacramento to Los Angeles, where we would change to a direct flight to Charles de Gaulle, we noticed the plane wasn't backing away from the gate. Soon came the announcement that an equipment problem would be delaying our takeoff. Tony and I realized we weren't going to make the Los Angeles flight to Paris if we continued to sit there.

3

While others onboard chatted about what was going on, we quickly got up, grabbed our carry-ons (all we ever take), and headed for the United Airlines check-in counter. Because we'd acted so swiftly, the agent was able to get us on a TWA flight about to depart for Saint Louis. From there, we could change to a nonstop TWA flight to Charles de Gaulle, arriving about the same time as we'd originally planned. Like characters on a TV commercial, we ran down the concourse to the TWA boarding gate, our carry-ons in tow. The flight had already boarded but they let us on.

Once off the ground, we praised ourselves. We'd been so much smarter than the other passengers. By the time we left the United Airlines counter with our TWA tickets in hand, those who'd been on the commuter flight had formed a long line behind us. Ah, pride. "Caution, caution," the Buddha would have said, but at that moment we were so pleased with ourselves for deftly averting a disastrous beginning to our special vacation. Several doctors have told us that the odds are high that on one of these two TWA flights I picked up the virus from which I have never recovered.

We arrived at our studio apartment on the tiny rue du Vieux Colombier in the sixth arrondissement on the Left Bank. The apartment was much smaller than it had looked in the online pictures. It consisted of a bathroom and a kitchen, each of which could be comfortably occupied by only one person at a time, and a living room. It was furnished with a tiny table and two chairs, a love seat (a romantic euphemism for a couch that's too small to lie down on), and a double bed in the corner. On the wall opposite the bed sat a bookshelf with a cabinet at the bottom. We found a tiny television set inside, but we had no intention of spending our time in Paris watching TV.

We wandered around that first day, waiting for nightfall so we could sleep and adjust to the new time zone. The next day,

I didn't feel well but assumed it was only jet lag. The day after that, I felt awful but, refusing to believe it could be anything other than lingering jet lag, I suggested we go to a movie. We picked an American film, *Anniversary Party*. Frankly, I just wanted to sit in the dark and try to assess what was going on in my body. While watching the movie, I began to realize that I was indeed sick.

Soon thereafter I developed typical flu symptoms and couldn't get out of bed. After three days, Tony and I reached the same hopeful conclusion: "This is no big deal. We still have eighteen days left in Paris."

After a week, it became "No big deal, we still have two weeks left in Paris."

". . . we still have ten days left in Paris."

The "days left" dwindled and dwindled.

We developed a routine. In the morning, Tony would go to a brasserie and then walk the streets of Paris, returning around noon, always hoping for a change in my condition. Then he'd go out in the afternoon for more walking. Maybe he would take in a museum. He was not enjoying these solo excursions.

During the second week of our stay, I wanted so badly to keep Tony company that I decided one day to tough it out. I insisted we go to see the famous Impressionist collection at the Musée d'Orsay, which had been converted from a train station into a museum and is known for its soaring interior spaces. The line to get in went around the block. We would have returned to the apartment right then and there had I not done my research and known to buy museum passes at a Métro station. Under the assumption we'd be museum-hopping together, Tony had bought two passes on our second day in Paris. We were allowed inside immediately.

As soon as I entered the Impressionist gallery, the adrenaline I'd used to get myself there wore off—this excursion had been a mistake. I collapsed into one of the lovely wicker chairs that sit in rows in the middle of the bigger galleries and told Tony to go ahead and enjoy the paintings. He would periodically come back and check on me, asking if we should leave, but I kept telling him to go off and look for a while longer.

As I sat, my eyes lit on a large painting by Claude Monet, *Essai de figure en plein-air: Femme à l'ombrelle tournée vers la droite.* A woman stands in a field, her face shaded by her umbrella. It's painted with a soft, muted palette, yet is somehow wonderfully luminous. I was vaguely aware of musical wicker chairs going on around me—people would sit for a few minutes, get up, and be quickly replaced by someone who had been waiting to take the first free chair. I just sat, bathed in the colors and the composition on Monet's canvas. I felt as if he'd painted this young woman in a field to watch over me so I could let Tony experience the museum. But my attempt at keeping him company had failed.

Except to see a doctor, that was the end of going out. My days were spent in bed. Too sick to read, I thought I'd try the little television after all. I was shocked at the poor quality of French programming: every channel had the worst kind of quiz show, featuring contestants who'd been coached to scream on cue, loud-mouthed obnoxious hosts, and the gaudiest of sets. In my naïveté, I was expecting high French culture to emanate from the tube. I gave up in frustration, but as the hours wore on, and I was still bored and restless, I tried TV again. I heard familiar theme music, actors were running around pushing a gurney, and on the screen the word *Emerges* appeared. Even with my poor French, I knew this was *ER*. I settled in for some televised comfort food, only to find it was dubbed into French. Movies in English were also dubbed instead of subtitled. "So much for TV," I thought, as I turned it off and closed the cabinet doors.

I spent most of each day and many a night when I was too sick to sleep listening to the BBC on a shortwave radio Tony bought for me when it was clear I'd be in bed for a while. The BBC had a wonderful array of programs, including clever and funny quiz shows. It became my introduction to our own National Public Radio (NPR), which I began listening to every day soon after returning to Davis and finding myself bedbound. When I'm listening to NPR's broadcast of the BBC News and I hear the plummy tones of the very same British voice that came over the shortwave radio in our Paris apartment announcing, "You're listening to the BBC World Service," a tinge of sadness passes over me. I'm briefly transported back to that bed on the Left Bank where it all began.

A few days after the trip to the Musée d'Orsay, we decided I should see a doctor. I looked in the yellow pages and found an entry for the "American Hospital." Even though the name suggested home and a refuge for me, the person who answered the phone was just plain rude. When I described my symptoms, she gruffly said, "Well, what do you want *us* to do about it?" It was a harbinger of things to come back in California.

Next I tried the entry for the "British Hospital." The woman who answered the phone only spoke French, but I heard concern and kindness in her voice. She put me on hold while she found a nurse who spoke English. She told me to come right in.

I still shake my head in disbelief when I think of the unnecessary stress we subjected ourselves to getting from our apartment on the Left Bank to the British hospital in a northern suburb of Paris, and thereafter to a pharmacy in central Paris, and then finally back to the Left Bank. Whew! Typical Californians, we never considered taking a cab. We weren't being cheap; it just didn't cross our minds. We think of cabs as something New Yorkers use. Foolishly, we walked from our apartment to the nearest Métro stop. Two transfers and several staircases later, we found ourselves above ground in an altogether different sort of Paris—the suburbs. Walking along with our map in hand, we made agonizingly slow progress. Even this small excursion was wearing me out.

The doctor thought I simply had the flu. She wrote down my diagnosis as *grippe*—a word that made me think of the rhyme for "postnasal drip" in Miss Adelaide's song from *Guys and Dolls*. She wanted to be sure it didn't turn into a bacterial infection that would ruin our whole vacation, so she gave me a prescription for antibiotics. We trekked back to the Métro and, after another transfer and more stairs, surfaced above ground at the only open pharmacy between the northern suburb and our Left Bank apartment, since it was one of those European days off intriguingly called a bank holiday.

The hospital and pharmacy ordeal is a haze in my mind, although a few vivid memories remain. I recall the hospital staff repeatedly apologizing because, since it was a bank holiday, they had to charge us for the appointment—a whopping fifteen dollars when converted from francs to dollars. I recall surfacing from the Métro to go to the pharmacy and finding myself face to face with a postcard-picture view of the Arc de Triomphe, the tiniest flash of the Paris we'd hoped to be seeing for three weeks. I also remember the agony I felt as I leaned against the wall in the Métro stairwells, using both hands on the banister to pull my body up step after step. Tony told me, years later, that when he saw me dragging my body up the stairs, he realized how sick I was. That's *his* vivid memory of that day.

Our last week in Paris, I turned on the TV again and discovered that the French Open was on all day long. Language didn't matter in tennis; even I could figure out that *égalité* meant "deuce." I made a bed for myself on the floor, close enough to the TV to be able to see the ball being hit over the net, and a love affair was born. I still watch a lot of tennis. I can recite the names of players from all over the world. I love how international tennis is. I love the aesthetics of the game—complexity within seeming simplicity. All a player has to do is get the ball over the net, inside the lines. But within that seeming simplicity lies an array of strategies— physical and mental—that has the feel of a chess game: aces, lobs, volleys, passing shots. As I lay there learning to love watching tennis, it seemed I might be getting better. I was deeply disappointed that our vacation had been ruined, but I was hopeful.

The day before we were scheduled to fly home, I felt I was on the road to recovery.

2

Staying Sick

THIS CAN'T BE HAPPENING TO ME

You can argue with the way things are.
You'll lose, but only 100% of the time.
—BYRON KATIE

A WEEK AFTER RETURNING, I had a relapse. Then once again, I seemed to get better except, strangely, my voice didn't return. This new whisper of a voice was troublesome because, as a teacher, I made my living by talking. In early July, with the law school semester starting at the end of August, I shared my concerns with the dean, but he was confident I'd be fine by then. We agreed not to worry.

In mid-July, feeling stronger and stronger, I went ahead with plans to go on a ten-day meditation retreat at Spirit Rock Meditation Center, in Marin County, north of San Francisco, about two hours from my home. This was a treasured annual retreat for Buddhist practitioners on the West Coast because the two principal teachers—Joseph Goldstein and Sharon Salzberg—had, along with Jack Kornfield, brought *vipassana* meditation to the United States after intensive training with teachers in Thailand,

Burma, and India. They founded the Insight Meditation Society (IMS) in Barre, Massachusetts, which instantly became a mecca for Americans who wanted to learn to meditate. Some years later, Jack moved to California and, along with other vipassana teachers, founded Spirit Rock.

Once a year, Joseph and Sharon, along with other IMS teachers, led a ten-day retreat at Spirit Rock, a retreat so popular that one could only get in through a lottery system. Except for my whisper of a voice, I appeared to be over what my primary care doctor now humorously called "the Parisian Flu." And, besides, one doesn't *need* a voice on a silent retreat. This year, Carol Wilson, Kamala Masters, and Steve Armstrong—all wonderful teachers—accompanied Joseph and Sharon. I thought, "Lucky, lucky me."

It was during this retreat that the Parisian Flu turned from acute to chronic. Eerily, I have it documented, although at the time I didn't know I was describing symptoms that would still be with me years and years later. I'd taken a notebook with me to jot down tidbits from the teachers' talks. It was not intended to be a daily diary, but what was happening to me was too curious not to keep track of. On Monday morning (the third day of the retreat), I wrote, "Woke up feeling sick. Am worried is same stuff again. Determined to stay here even if can only go to teachers' talks."

That night, I wrote, "Feel as if I'm in a stupor. Have this humming, angry pulsating feeling in the body as if I've been up for several nights, not like any other illness I've ever had."

On Tuesday, I wrote, "Definitely sick. What's going on? Very confused."

Determined to stay at the retreat, at one point I wrote, "If one is to be sick and alone, this is as good a place as any." But aside from attending a few talks (there was one each evening) and going to the eating hall once a day for lunch because wiping down the tables afterward was my work meditation, I stayed in my room. Since the residence halls are up a steep hill from the eating hall, I wrote, "Coming up the hill, I feel like I'm coming up the stairs in the Métro. The flashback is vivid."

Although I felt too sick to sit up and meditate, I tried to follow a basic meditation instruction: watch the mind. "Worry is arising," I wrote. A neutral, nonattached observation of fact. But I couldn't maintain that meditative perspective for long, and so "Worry is arising" was soon followed by an outpouring of troubled thoughts and questions: "Did they read a blood test wrong?. . . I would like to absorb into TV. . . . In my room and sad, second-guessing if I should go home to see the doctor. So sad. So sad, especially since I now know the joy of being well."

I didn't go back to work at the end of August in 2001. The dean found someone to cover my classes. I also didn't get to spend time with my new granddaughter, Malia, whose first year of life was going by fast. That fall, my life was spent in bed or at a doctor's office. I entered the phase of the illness in which we needed to rule out every cause that could show up in blood tests, CT scans, MRIs, and other procedures, some of which were completely foreign to me (such as the painful but fascinating appointment at which a technician made a videotape of my voice box to be examined for abnormalities).

I had so much blood drawn that we joked with my primary care doctor that at least we'd proven that bloodletting didn't appear to be a cure. I was referred to half a dozen specialists. All I could tell them was that I had flu-like symptoms without the fever; an extremely hoarse voice; eighteen pounds of weight loss; and a fatigue so devastating that, no matter how small the waiting-room chair, I tried to turn it into a bed.

In the end, I saw three infectious disease doctors; two ear, nose, and throat specialists; a rheumatologist, an endocrinologist, a gastroenterologist, a neurologist, a cardiologist, and (on my own) two acupuncturists. Each ran his or her own battery of tests. Even though I was never referred to an oncologist, I still found myself at my medical provider's cancer center because the endocrinologist wanted to test my adrenal function using an infusion test that could only be performed at the clinic where cancer patients received chemotherapy. I met some brave people that day.

All the tests indicated that nothing was wrong with me. So in the spring of 2002, I dragged myself back to the law school twice a week to teach a class that met for ninety minutes each session. I went back to work mainly because I simply could not and would not believe I wasn't going to get better. Everyone I saw at work assumed I'd finally recovered. After all, I didn't look sick to them. They would stop me in the hall to chat, seemingly unaware that I was leaning against the wall to keep from falling over.

I continued to work part-time for two and a half years, sometimes going to the law school twice a week, sometimes three times a week, depending on the class schedule. Even though Tony worked in another town, he tried to arrange his schedule so he could drive me the ten minutes from our house to the law school and pick me up after my class. I was too sick to drive myself ten minutes to work, yet I'd teach a class that sometimes lasted an hour and a half.

It's easy to look back and see what a mistake it was to continue working while sick—it probably worsened my condition—but many people who are chronically ill have done the same. First, there's the financial need to keep working. Second, there's the utter disbelief that this is happening to you (reinforced by people telling you that you look fine—people who don't see you collapse on the bed as soon as you get home). Each morning, you expect to wake up *not feeling sick* even though for weeks and then months—and then years—that has never been the case. It's just so

14   *How Everything Changed*

hard to, first, truly recognize that you're chronically ill and, second, accept that this illness is going to require you to change your plans for life in ways you never imagined, not the least of which is giving up the career you loved and worked so hard to build.

I had to come up with secret coping mechanisms to make it through my part-time workday. For the first time in twenty years, I took a chair into the classroom and taught while sitting down. The noise made by lively chatting students, as many as eighty at a time, was so jarring to my sick body that I wore ear plugs as I entered the room, then discreetly removed them as the students quieted down for me to begin talking. I concocted a method to keep students from coming to my office because, once I was in there with them, I lost the ability to control the length of the interaction. If someone approached me after class and another class was following mine in the same room, I'd find an empty classroom and sit down there with the student. That way, when I felt I'd answered his or her questions, I could stand up and end the conversation.

I even had a secret coping technique I didn't tell Tony about because it felt too deviant. My office wasn't close to a bathroom. Not only was I too sick to walk to the bathroom on the other side of the building, but in doing so I risked running into colleagues who might (with the best of intentions) want to engage me in conversation while standing in the hallway. Avoiding those encounters was among my highest priorities. So I found an old thermos and took it to my office. I peed into it, screwed the lid on tightly, put it in my bag, and took it home to empty and wash out.

Those who have no choice but to go to work while chronically ill all have secret coping mechanisms. At first I felt humiliated having to use subterfuges and to undergo such indignity just to relieve myself. I blamed myself for my life having brought me to this sorry state. After a while the self-loathing shifted to a defiant but ugly cynicism: healthy people be damned; this is what I'm doing, so shove it if you don't approve. Fortunately, the cynicism gave way to compassion for myself. If nothing else, peeing into a thermos was no easy feat: I was professionally dressed for class, pantyhose and all.

I never told the students I was sick (although some of them figured it out). However, being sick, I was unable to be anyone other than my unadorned self in the classroom. It became easy to admit that I didn't know the answer to a question. I spoke in such a weak voice that students sometimes had to ask me to repeat myself. This experience gave me a new compassion both for people caught up in the legal system and for students facing struggles in their personal lives.

Even as I sat in a chair, even as I felt myself struggle, I received the highest teaching evaluations in my twenty years on the job. And yet I couldn't sustain the effort. When you are as sick as I am, you have to make some very tough choices. I had to let it all go. Ironically, people may think you're giving up, when in fact you are simply giving in to the reality of your new life.

For me, that reality meant having the symptoms that accompany a severe flu, including the dazed sick feeling and the aches and pains, but without the fever, the sore throat, or the cough. To imagine it, multiply the fatigue and the aches and pains of the flu by an order of magnitude. Add in a heart that's constantly pounding with the kind of wired, oppressive fatigue that healthy people associate with severe jet lag, making it hard to concentrate or even watch TV—let alone nap or sleep at night.

Part of the reality for many who suffer from chronic debilitating illnesses is the continuing quest to try to figure out why we are so sick and in pain—and never getting a definitive answer. If being labeled with an acronym could cure me, I'd be in great shape. Since getting sick in Paris, I've been diagnosed with a laundry list of diseases and conditions: CFS (aka CFIDS, ME, ME/CFS), PVS,

VICD, OI, POTS, PEM, and SEID. (If you'd like to know what these letters and various diagnoses mean, see the box below.)

In the end, though, all we really know is this: I got sick on a trip to Paris and I never got well. But I also began a journey into the depths of the Buddha's teaching. I needed to learn how to be sick.

How do you name my illness? Let me count the ways.

Chronic Fatigue Syndrome. CFS is the name of my diagnosis that most people are familiar with. Unfortunately, it's terribly misleading and trivializes a serious disease. First, what illness isn't fatiguing? What *day* isn't fatiguing? Second, take my word for it, the word *fatigue* doesn't begin to describe how I feel every day. When people are given this diagnosis, it's not uncommon for family, friends, and even the medical community to dismiss the sufferer as being nothing more than tired.

Chronic Fatigue and Immune Dysfunction Syndrome. CFIDS is an alternative name given to CFS, partially in an attempt to have it taken seriously and partially because a subset of CFS patients (including me) appear to have an overactive immune system that produces flu-like symptoms due to the body remaining in a perpetual state of "sickness response."

Myalgic Encephalomyelitis. Myalgic encephalomyelitis (ME) is the name given to this illness in almost every country except the United States, Canada, and Australia. Myalgic encephalomyelitis has become the preferred name among most patient advocates; in the United States, there's been some progress in getting the name changed from CFS to ME. Throughout the book, I'll refer to the illness as ME/CFS because that's the most common designation as of this writing.

Post-Viral Syndrome. A few decades ago the Centers for Disease Control (CDC) rejected the name PVS in favor of CFS. Some doctors still use the name and did so with me, especially in the first two years following the Parisian Flu.

Viral Induced Central Nervous System Dysfunction. VICD is a fairly recent designation, used to describe a subset of ME/CFS patients whose blood work indicates there may be a reactivation of herpes viruses that usually lie dormant in the body after their acute childhood phases. My bloodwork suggests that I fit this subset, although antivirals haven't helped me. The theory is that an acute infection—in my case, the Parisian Flu—triggers a reactivation of the viruses, causing the immune system to become engaged in a constant low-grade war against them.

Orthostatic Intolerance and Postural Tachycardia Syndrome. These two diagnoses refer to poor blood circulation, which makes it difficult to maintain a standing position. They are thought to be results of whatever is wrong with ME/CFS sufferers as opposed to the cause.

Post-Exertional Malaise. One characteristic of ME/CFS is its great range of symptoms. I've met dozens of people on the Internet who have been diagnosed with ME/CFS, and none of us have all the same symptoms. Some have chronic sore throats and swollen lymph glands. Others (like me) do not but suffer from an unremitting flu-like malaise. Some experience cognitive impairment, including difficulty processing information, forgetfulness, and an inability to form sentences properly. Others (like me) do not, except to the extent that flu-like symptoms make it hard to concentrate. Some (like me) suffer from muscle and joint pain. Others do not. The only symptom that everyone with this diagnosis shares is post-exertional malaise (PEM). This refers to an exacerbation of symptoms following either physical or mental activity even though these activities were easily tolerated before the onset of the illness. PEM can cause a person to become bedbound for days or for weeks.

Systemic Exertion Intolerance Disease. In 2014, the United States Department of Health and Human Services, along with the CDC, the Food and Drug Administration, and several other agencies, asked the Institute of Medicine (IOM, now called the National Academy of Medicine) to appoint a committee of experts to examine the evidence base for ME/CFS. The IOM committee concluded that ME/CFS is a serious, chronic, complex, systemic disease that can profoundly affect the lives of patients. The committee recommended that the name be changed to systemic exertion intolerance disease (SEID) because that designation best describes the one symptom that all sufferers have in common: PEM. So far, the name SEID has not caught on.

I'm convinced, as are many experts, that ME/CFS represents several discrete illnesses. It's disheartening and unacceptable that the government allocates so little research funding to study this illness. Until this changes, little progress will be made in finding a cause or a cure. It remains a tragedy for millions of people and their families.

Pain Is Part of Life

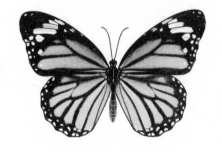

3

The Buddha Tells It Like It Is

To go into the dark with a light is to know the light.
To know the dark, go dark. Go without sight
and find that the dark, too, blooms and sings,
and is traveled by dark feet and dark wings.
—WENDELL BERRY

AFTER A LONG journey of discovery, with many ups and downs, the Buddha, an ordinary human being like you and me, sat down under a tree and stayed there until he attained enlightenment—also known as liberation, freedom, or awakening. At first he wasn't sure if he could find the words to share his experience, but eventually he gave his first teaching in the form of what is known as the Four Noble Truths. Buddhism—what Buddhists call the Dharma, which means "teachings"—was born.

The Buddha's List

Many people will tell you they know the first noble truth, but their usual rendering, "Life is suffering," is responsible for a lot of misunderstanding about what the Buddha taught. In offering

23

us the first noble truth, the Buddha was not making a negative pronouncement. He was describing the conditions of life that are shared by all human beings. He presented them as a list of experiences that all of us, including the Buddha, can expect to encounter at one time or another during our lifetimes: birth, aging, illness, death, sorrow, pain, grief, getting what we don't want, not getting what we want, and losing what we cherish.

Notice that illness is on the list, meaning that it's a natural part of the human life cycle. How many people think of illness as natural? I hadn't—until I encountered the Buddha's list.

What all the items have in common is that none of them are pleasant experiences; indeed, they are often mentally painful or physically painful. It's a daunting list, that's for sure. No wonder people sometimes say that Buddhism is pessimistic. It's not to me, though. The Buddha was simply being realistic and honest about the human condition. Since all of us will face these experiences at one time or another during our lives, I appreciate that the Buddha was upfront about them so I can start, right now, learning to respond wisely when they occur.

As I understand the Buddha's intent, he began his teachings with these unpleasant and often painful experiences because we spend so much time in a fruitless effort to deny their presence or to try to make them go away. It is this relentless effort to escape what we cannot escape and to change what we cannot change that leads us to be dissatisfied with our lives.

The word the Buddha used to describe this dissatisfaction is *dukkha*. It comes from Pali, the language in which the Buddha's teachings were first recorded.

Dukkha is too multifaceted and nuanced a term to be captured in its usual one-word translation, "suffering." To capture the essence of what the Buddha meant by the presence of dukkha in

24   *Pain Is Part of Life*

our lives, it's helpful to keep other possible translations of this key word in mind: unsatisfactoriness (that is, dissatisfaction with the circumstances of our lives), anguish, stress, discomfort, unease, to name a few. Dukkha is a term worth becoming familiar with, especially when exploring how to be sick.

When I first encountered the various translations for dukkha, they resonated powerfully for me. Finally, someone was describing this life in a way that fit a good portion of my experience, both physical and mental: stress, discomfort, unsatisfactoriness. What a relief to know it wasn't just *me* and wasn't just *my* life!

The feeling that the Buddha understood the difficulties I faced allowed me to start the day-to-day work of making peace with the realization that unpleasant and painful experiences are part of the human condition, and that we create dukkha—suffering, stress, anguish—when we resist this. Even in the darkest early days of the illness, when I didn't understand what was happening to me (was I dying?), I always had the first noble truth propping me up, telling me, "You know this is the way it is. You were born and so are subject to illness. It happens differently for each person. This is one of the ways it's happening to you."

The Buddha didn't say that life is *only* made up of the unpleasant experiences on his list. He was simply emphasizing that difficulties are present in the life of all human beings. Years ago, a law student told me that Buddhism was pessimistic. When I asked him why he thought that, he said, "Well, the first noble truth is 'Life sucks.'" In trying to explain to him why that was not a valid translation of the Buddha's teaching, a shift occurred in how I thought of the first noble truth.

Yes, it's true that life brings with it a considerable share of unpleasantness and difficulties, but happiness and joy are available, too. The fourth-century B.C.E. Taoist sage Chuang Tzu referred to this world, this life we're living right now, as the realm of the ten thousand joys and the ten thousand sorrows. The Buddha began his teachings by focusing on the ten thousand sorrows because our inability to accept them as part of life only makes things harder for us.

It's a challenge to make peace with the Buddha's list. This is partly because we've evolved to seek pleasant experiences and to avoid unpleasant ones. After all, doing so might be crucial to our survival; if we were living in the wild and didn't run fast from some unpleasant experiences, we'd have ended up as some animal's dinner! In our modern world, however, this bias to continually seek what's pleasant and react with aversion to what's unpleasant doesn't always serve us well.

The first noble truth helps me gracefully accept being chronically ill. The Buddha's list assures me that my life is as it should be because it's unfolding in accord with the human condition, difficult as that can be at times. "Our life is always all right," says the Zen teacher Charlotte Joko Beck in *Everyday Zen*. "There's nothing wrong with it. Even if we have horrendous problems, it's just our life." Her words resonate powerfully for me every time I read them.

For me, "just my life" has meant ending my professional career years before I expected to, being housebound and even bedbound much of the time, feeling continually sick and often in pain, and living with the anxiety that pops up now and then that the cancer might return. Using Joko Beck's words, I've been able to take these facts that make up my life as a starting point—to bow down to them and to accept them. From there, I work on looking around to see what life has to offer.

And I've found a lot.

The End of Dukkha

In the second noble truth, the Buddha said that what gives rise to dukkha is a specific type of desire I often refer to as "Want/Don't-Want Mind." The Buddha referred to this unskillful desire as "the unquenchable thirst." We experience it as an intense wanting—even a felt need—to have only pleasant experiences and not to have unpleasant ones. But neither of these two desires can be satisfied because they don't reflect the realities of the human condition.

When we react to life's unpleasant experiences by launching a militant battle against them—for example, by denying that we're chronically ill or by turning away in aversion from the need to grieve our losses—we create dukkha (suffering, stress, dissatisfaction). We also create dukkha when we expect to have only pleasant experiences, even though no one's life is pleasant all the time. In short, when we're unable to accept that our lives will be a mixture of joys and sorrows, pleasantness and unpleasantness, successes and disappointments, we make things worse for ourselves because we're adding dukkha to the mix.

In the third noble truth, the Buddha proclaimed that the end of dukkha is possible. It's important to note, though, that bodily pain and suffering are an inescapable part of the human condition. Everyone experiences them at some point in life. The good news is that we *can* reach the end of suffering in the mind—even while in this suffering body.

In the fourth noble truth, the Buddha set out the lesson plan to accomplish this: the Eightfold Path. Most of the elements on this path make an appearance in this book. Wise understanding, which refers to seeing the truth of the human condition so we know what to expect in life, is the subject of this chapter and the two that follow. Wise intention—which manifests as kindness, compassion, empathetic joy, and calm abiding—is the subject of chapters 6 through 9. Also covered are wise speech, wise action, wise mindfulness (keeping ourselves in the present moment), and wise effort (effort that helps alleviate suffering in ourselves and others).

With the end of dukkha comes enlightenment, awakening, liberation, freedom—I suggest you pick a word that resonates best with you. We may not be able to complete the lesson plan of the Eightfold Path in this life; we may not become fully enlightened beings any time soon. That said, a glimpse of awakening, a moment of liberation, a taste of freedom is available to us all—and it can take us a long way toward easing our experience of dukkha.

4

The Universal Law of Impermanence

Better a single day of life
seeing the reality of arising and passing away
than a hundred years of existence remaining blind to it.
—THE BUDDHA

A CRUCIAL STEP ON the path to freedom and peace of mind is understanding what the Buddha called "the three marks of experience"—three experiences that are common to the life of every human being. We looked at the first mark—dukkha—in the previous chapter. The other two are impermanence (*anicca*) and no-fixed-self (*anatta*). They're the subjects of this chapter and the next one, respectively.

Impermanence is recognized as a universal law in other spiritual traditions and in science as well. At a Spirit Rock retreat in the late 1990s, Joseph Goldstein gave what has become my favorite description of impermanence as I experience it in everyday life: "Anything can happen at any time."

Initially I reacted to his statement the same way I reacted when I first encountered the Buddha's teaching that everything is impermanent; I thought, "Yeah, tell me something I *don't* know." But

29

when I didn't recover my health, I began to deeply contemplate the meaning of "anything can happen at any time"—such as getting sick and not getting better, such as having to give up my profession, such as rarely being able to leave the house. Yes, anything *can* happen at any time.

How are we to find any solace in this universal law? The thirteenth-century Zen master Dogen offers a clue in the *Eihei Koroku*:

> Without the bitterest cold that penetrates to the very bone, how can plum blossoms send forth their fragrance all over the universe?

When we begin to see the truth of impermanence, there's a tendency to focus on Dogen's "the bitterest cold that penetrates to the very bone." Having had to give up my profession still feels like that on some days. The challenge becomes finding the fragrance sent forth by those plum blossoms. Without the bitter cold of being bedbound most of the day, I wouldn't be so attuned to the changing seasons; I never realized they are on view right outside my bedroom window. Without the bitter cold of having to give up my profession, I wouldn't have discovered the joy of growing trees in my bedroom. (Yes, bonsai, but trees nonetheless!) I return to Dogen's verse over and over for inspiration.

The writings of the Vietnamese Zen master Thich Nhat Hanh have also helped me see the beauty inherent in the fact of impermanence. In his biography of the Buddha, *Old Path White Clouds,* Thich Nhat Hanh points out that impermanence is the very condition necessary for life. Without it, nothing could grow or develop. A grain of rice could not grow into a rice plant; a child could not grow into an adult. There are so many ways in which I've "grown" only because of this illness, from a heightened awareness and compassion for the chronically ill and those who care for them, to a deep appreciation for the hard-working people who go unnoticed but keep our infrastructure running. (I see them from my house—delivering mail, climbing power poles, cleaning the streets—whether it's over a hundred degrees outside or pouring rain.)

Uncertainty and Unpredictability

With impermanence comes uncertainty and unpredictability. These two characteristics of the human condition can be a deep source of anxiety and stress for us because we crave the opposite: security and assurance. We wish we could control what happens to us. If we could, life would never be difficult or painful. We'd make sure of that by ordering up only pleasant experiences. "Body: feel good all the time, and don't get old! Mind: get calm, and I mean *now*!" Has barking orders at yourself ever worked for you?

We control much less of our experience than we realize. Not only do we lack the control we'd like to have over our bodies and our minds, but we also don't control what's going on around us—from how people treat us to the tragedies and violent conflicts around the world. Recall the second noble truth and how our Want/Don't-Want Mind operates. We want pleasant experiences and we don't want unpleasant ones. We want people and the world to conform to our wishes, and we don't want to feel that we lack control of our bodies and our minds.

Here's one way to work on coming to terms with life's uncertainty and unpredictability. First, with kindness and compassion, gently acknowledge that we're not sure how our lives will unfold and that this can feel mightily uncomfortable—even scary—at times. Second, work on keeping our attention in the present moment so as to avoid spinning and feeding stressful stories and scenarios about a future we cannot predict anyway. The more we're able to do this, the less we'll suffer.

Weather Practice

Here I offer a practice to help us make peace with life's uncertainty and unpredictability; I call it "weather practice." It was inspired by, of all things, the 2005 movie *The Weather Man*, starring Nicolas Cage as a character named Dave Spritz.

Dave is adrift in life, even though he has a steady job as the weatherman for a Chicago TV station. In reality he's just a "weather reader," dependent on a meteorologist to tell him what to say. When the meteorologist gives him a forecast with an eighteen-degree variance, Dave complains that he needs something more concrete. The meteorologist responds, "Dave, it's random. We do our best." One day the meteorologist preps Dave for his TV spot by saying, "We might see some snow, but it might shift south and miss us." When Dave protests that the viewers will want a more certain forecast than that, the meteorologist tells him that predicting the weather is a guess. "It's wind, man," he says. "It blows all over the place."

I found this amusing at the time, but it's turned out to be extremely useful in life. When uncertainty and unpredictability throw me for a loop, I like to say to Tony, "Here it is again, life and the weather. Just wind, man, blowing all over the place." Then returning to the verse from Dogen, I remind myself that the wind that's blowing the bitterest cold at me may be setting the stage for something joyful to follow.

I work on treating thoughts and moods as wind, blowing into the mind and blowing out. We can't control what thoughts arise in the mind. (Telling yourself not to think about whether you'll feel well enough to join the family for dinner is almost a guarantee that it's exactly what you *will* think about!) And moods are as uncontrollable as thoughts. Blue moods arise uninvited, as does fear or anxiety. By working with this wind metaphor, I can hold painful thoughts and blue moods more lightly, knowing they'll blow on through soon—after all, that's what they do. Here are two examples of Weather Practice in action.

One night I felt so sick that I wanted to throw out all the work I'd done on this book. Dark thoughts. A blue mood. My eyes welled up with tears. But instead of those tears turning into sobs, I took a deep breath and began this weather practice, remembering that thoughts and moods blow all over the place and that if I just waited, these particular ones would blow on through. And they did.

When it became clear that the Parisian Flu had settled into a chronic illness, Tony and I began to consider if it was feasible for him to go on a retreat for an entire month during which he'd be out of contact with me unless I called with an emergency. I badly wanted him to go because I saw it as a way I could feel like a caregiver for him. He went for the first time in 2005 and each February thereafter. The retreat became a major annual event for him. The preparations he made ahead of time were like those that people make who are in the path of a coming hurricane. He brought a month of supplies into the house. He filled the freezer with food he'd cooked ahead of time. He set up people in town for me to contact if I needed help. My promise to him was to be extra careful in everything I did and to call him home if I needed him.

The forecast inside our house for February 2009 called for "calm weather" despite my illness. But at nine A.M., two days after Tony left, things changed in a split second. One moment I was at the top of the two steps that lead down to our bedroom; the next moment I was writhing in pain on the bedroom floor, having slipped down the steps and landed on my right ankle.

When the pain began to subside, I pulled myself up on the bed and went straight to my laptop to research the only question on my mind: Was I going to have to go to the doctor? Medical appointments can be an ordeal for the chronically ill—the round-trip drive, the possibility of a long wait, the energy it takes to effectively communicate with the doctor. It's so much easier to have a caregiver along. When I go to the doctor, Tony drives me, stands in line to check in for me, and accompanies me to the examining room. I never schedule medical appointments during February.

Despite the rapidly increasing swelling and discoloration on my ankle, my Internet research convinced me that I only needed to go to the doctor if I still couldn't put weight on it in twenty-four hours. So I waited. When I needed to go somewhere off the bed, I crawled. Our dog, Rusty, acted as if I'd finally seen the light and was joining his species. This appeared to be a cause for great celebration for him, so my added challenge became to make sure that in his exuberance he didn't step on my right foot.

That first day, as I lay in pain on the bed, I thought of the meteorologist's comment to Dave the weather reader: "Dave, it's random. We do our best." Tony and I had indeed done our best to prepare for a calm February, but, as we all discover again and again, anything can happen at any time. We can take precautions, but predicting the future is as futile as predicting which way the wind will blow.

The next morning, when I still couldn't put weight on my right foot, our friend Richard took me to the doctor. Diagnosis: fractured fibula. The forecast: no weight bearing on it for several weeks; a cast so heavy that it took all my energy to move my leg; crutches and crawling to get around. I toughed it out for one more day. Even with people offering to help, the injury on top of the illness proved to be too much. One or the other I could have

34   *Pain Is Part of Life*

handled alone but not both. I knew I needed to call Tony home when, before going to sleep for the night, it took me ten minutes to negotiate a trip to the bathroom even though it's only footsteps from the bed. After making one round trip, I lay back on the bed in exhaustion and then realized that the light over the bathroom sink was still on—a light that shines right in my eyes. I had no choice but to start the process of getting to the bathroom and back all over again.

So Tony came home four days into his treasured month-long retreat and, for a month, traded his caregiver role for that of nursemaid. Life and the weather—one moment it's calm and the next moment a nasty storm has blown in.

Weather practice is a powerful reminder of the fleeting nature of experience, how each moment arises and passes as quickly as a weather pattern. A week after I fell, I went to see an orthopedic surgeon. My regular doctor arranged the consult in case I needed surgery to insert a plate and pins. A resident came into the examining room first. Looking at the x-rays, he said that, given the nature of the break and the damage to the ligaments, I might very well need surgery to stabilize the area. He left the room to report his findings to the orthopedic surgeon—and dark storm clouds gathered as Tony and I contemplated the effect on my illness if I had to go through surgery. I was expecting heavy rain to accompany the surgeon into the room, but he walked in and immediately said, "Surgery? No, no, no! The area is stable. You just need to stay off the ankle as long as it hurts and get physical therapy to regain your range of motion." In a flash, the sun had burst through the clouds. Tony and I were elated.

But a half-hour later, as I lay on the bed trying to nap, a cold dense fog settled in as I thought, "What does it matter that the surgeon gave us such good news? Even when I can walk normally again, I'll still be sick and bedbound most of the day and

The Universal Law of Impermanence   35

Tony, despite all this extra care he's giving me, still won't have my company out there in the world." In a little over an hour, I'd experienced dark storm clouds, the threat of rain, the sun bursting through instead, and now a cold dense fog. Recognizing the fleeting nature of each moment, I was able to smile and the final verse of the *Diamond Sutra* came to mind:

> Thus shall you think of all this fleeting world:
> A star at dawn, a bubble in a stream;
> A flash of lightning in a summer cloud,
> A flickering lamp, a phantom, and a dream.

I knew it wouldn't be long before the sun would burn off that cold dense fog and I'd smell the fragrance of Dogen's plum blossoms.

Broken-Glass Practice

Finally, to help me live gracefully with the truth of uncertainty and unpredictability, I rely on what I call "broken-glass practice." This practice was inspired by a passage in *Food for the Heart*, a collection of teachings from the Thai Buddhist monk Ajahn Chah. He trained many Westerners at his remote forest monastery and has had a strong influence on the shape that Buddhism of South Asia has taken in the West. As we shall see in more detail later, he offers powerful teachings on equanimity: the ability to greet whatever is present in our experience with an evenness of temper, so that our minds stay balanced and steady in the face of life's ups and downs.

Here is Ajahn Chah talking about a glass:

> You say, "Don't break my glass!" Can you prevent something that's breakable from breaking? It will break

sooner or later. If you don't break it, someone else will. If someone else doesn't break it, one of the chickens will! . . . Penetrating the truth of these things, [we see] that this glass is already broken. . . . [The Buddha] saw the broken glass within the unbroken one. Whenever you use this glass, you should reflect that it's already broken. Whenever its time is up, it will break. Use the glass, look after it, until the day when it slips out of your hand and shatters. No problem. Why not? Because you saw its brokenness before it broke!

I use broken-glass practice all the time. The Buddha taught that all that arises is subject to change, decay, and dissolution. So when Tony or I break something, or the power goes off, or the landline goes dead because the neighborhood squirrels have been chewing on the wires again, we try to laugh and say, "Ah, it was already broken."

As a metaphor, broken-glass practice has helped me accept one of the consequences of being chronically ill—one that my online wanderings tell me would show up on the "top ten most difficult adjustments" list of most people who are sick or in mental or physical pain: the same activities that used to bring us the greatest joy are now the very activities that make our condition worse. This was a bitter pill for me to swallow; it still is sometimes.

These activities include everything from holiday dinners to special events, such as weddings. Having to sit upright for extended periods, trying to focus on a conversation while the room is full of noise, not feeling we can leave (or not having the means to leave) even though our bodies are crying out for us to lie down—these are but a few of the features of these activities that exacerbate the physical symptoms of the chronically ill. People who struggle with mental illness face similar challenges; imagine the toll on someone who has developed social anxiety but still must attend multiple winter holiday parties. Even someone in good health is likely to be mentally and physically exhausted after several of these gatherings, so it's not surprising that they can have such a devastating effect on those who are already chronically ill.

To me, broken-glass practice is particularly helpful in these situations. A guide at the end of the book lists several additional practices that can help us adjust to this most difficult aspect of impermanence—a change in our lives that keeps us from participating in or enjoying activities that we may have counted among our greatest joys. I find comfort in contemplating that my ability to participate in these activities was already broken, in the sense that this change in my life will befall everyone at some point and quite possibly by surprise. This is simply how and when it happened to me.

Then I reflect on impermanence—the fact that every aspect of my life is uncertain, unpredictable, and in constant flux. Finally, like Ajahn Chah, I look after each moment, cherishing what I still *can* do, aware that everything could change in an instant.

5

Who Is Sick? Who Is in Pain?

*What I am, as system theorists have helped me see,
is a "flow-through." I am a flow-through
of matter, energy, and information.*

—JOANNA MACY

BEFORE BECOMING CHRONICALLY ILL, I had the good fortune of attending several retreats at Spirit Rock co-led by the Theravadan teacher Kamala Masters. At one retreat, she told us a story about her root teacher, Munindra-ji, who lived in India.

Munindra-ji had always wanted to see the Buddhist sacred sites. He was getting quite old, so Kamala traveled to India with some friends to take him to some of the sites. One day they were waiting in a train station. The train was five hours late. It was blazing hot. They had no food. There were no restrooms. The platform where they were to catch the train kept changing, so they had to keep getting up and moving. Munindra-ji would sit down in each new location and rest his head on his arm. He looked so frail that Kamala began to worry about how he was holding up, especially since she and her friends were barely coping with the conditions. She finally asked him if he was all right. He replied,

"There is heat here, but I am not hot. There is hunger here, but I am not hungry. There is irritation here, but I am not irritated."

I recalled Kamala's story one day as I lay in bed after becoming sick, so I silently said, "There is sickness here, but I am not sick." The statement made no sense to me. But, inspired by the story, I persevered, repeating over and over, "There is sickness here, but I am not sick. There is sickness here, but I am not sick." After a few minutes, I realized, "Of course! There is sickness in the body, but *I* am not sick!"

It was a revelation and a source of great comfort. After a time, however, I decided to investigate more deeply. When I did, this question arose: "Who is this 'I' who isn't sick?" This question led me to consider the most radical implication of the universal law of impermanence—that what I think of as my "self" is also in constant flux. This is what the Buddha called the third mark of experience—anatta—which is usually translated as "no-self" or "no-fixed-self," depending on the context. It is the principal way in which he broke from the religion of his birth, Hinduism.

Of course, to communicate with others we have to use conventional terminology such as "I Me Mine" (to borrow from the title of the George Harrison song from *Let It Be*). If I'm unwilling to use the term *Toni Bernhard*, I can't get a driver's license or a disability check. And, as this very paragraph illustrates, I'll continue to use self-referential terms in this book. But I can use the word *I* and, even as the word emerges from the mind, still contemplate questions such as "Who am I? What is Toni Bernhard? Is Toni Bernhard a solid physical and mental entity with an inherent self-existence, or is Toni Bernhard a label attached to an ever-changing constellation of qualities?"

When people are first introduced to this teaching, some find it perplexing, some are even disturbed by it. I hope, like me, you find it worth investigating.

We all have a vague or even specific sense of "I am." It is this sense that leads the mind to imagine the existence of a permanent, unchanging self or identity around which our whole life revolves. Joseph Goldstein and Jack Kornfield express this beautifully in *Seeking the Heart of Wisdom*:

> Just as we condition our bodies in different ways through exercise or lack of it, so we also condition our minds. Every mind state, thought, or emotion that we experience repeatedly becomes stronger and more habituated. Who we are as personalities is a collection of all the tendencies of mind that have been developed, the particular energy configurations we have cultivated.

Consider who you were ten years ago. The part of your personality that seems to be consistent from then until now results not from any permanent entity carrying over from one moment to the next but from each moment being conditioned by the previous one. You cannot identify a permanent self that has carried over from ten years ago until now. "I" is a thought and a feeling, held on to so resolutely that the experience of a fixed person appears to be real.

Think of a bicycle. It's a temporary assemblage of steel, plastic, and human intelligence in a particular combination we conveniently designate "bicycle." There is no inherent "bikeness." It is the same with humans. There is no immutable, unchanging personality ("Toni Bernhard") that exists as an entity separate from the arising and passing of physical and mental activity—activity that is conditioned by preceding causes. No phenomenon—mental or physical—exists separate and independent from the conditions that give rise to it. This view is in contrast to religions that posit an immutable, eternal being or spiritual essence that is beyond cause and effect. As Steven Collins says in *Selfless Persons*, "There is nothing more to the 'person' but a temporary assemblage of parts."

Contemplating the truth of no-fixed-self has helped me tremendously since I became chronically ill. Haven't we all at some time thought, "If I could only get away from myself!"? Intuitively we know what a relief it would be to take I Me Mine out of the equation. (George Harrison's voice gently reminds us of the unremitting presence of "selfing" when he sings, "Even those tears, *I me mine, I me mine, I me mine.*") Experiencing no-self lifts a burden and brings a sense of spaciousness and freedom to everyday life.

Looking deeply at impermanence can help us experience no-self. Joseph Goldstein said during a retreat I attended that the mind and the body feel substantial, set, and solid, but if we watch carefully, there's nothing to hold on to. "Where's the mood you were in five minutes ago?" he asked. "Where's the thought of a few seconds ago? Where's that expert knowing self of two hours ago?" He suggested the answer was, "Gone!" When I contemplated his words, I understood that the mood, the thought, the expert were just momentary arisings in the mind.

Joseph went on to explain that we take these momentary arisings and string them together and soon they feel like something solid. Again, I contemplated this. "Ah, yes," I thought. "I string my thoughts together and then feel like the fixed entity 'Toni Bernhard.'" He asked us to see if we could control this fixed entity by issuing commands such as "Let me only have pleasant moods!" or "Let me not have this aching back!" I tried but could not get the mind or the body to obey these commands. What happens in life arises out of conditions, not from a "me" in control.

I like to purposefully think "I am Toni Bernhard" and then contemplate if this is true. People *call* me "Toni Bernhard" and I respond when they do. (I get up from the waiting-room chair at the doctor's office when those two words are called out!) But I can find no fixed, unchanging, permanent entity. There is no Toni Bernhard. And that's fine. Life is an unfolding process and will take whatever course it takes.

Contemplating the perennial question "Who am I?" can also help us experience no-self. This question is a tool used by Western philosophers and Eastern mystics alike, although their answers to the question may differ. For example, in *The Only Dance There Is*, spiritual teacher Ram Dass discusses the difference in the Western and Eastern approaches to this question. He compares Descartes's "I think, therefore I am" with the more no-self-flavored formulation, "I think, but I am not my thoughts."

While in India in 1967, Richard Alpert became a disciple of the Hindu sage Neem Karoli Baba, who gave him the name Ram Dass. Neem Karoli Baba didn't give formal discourses. He told stories and sometimes spoke only a few words to a disciple before sending him or her away. Many years ago, I read an interview with Ram Dass in which he said that when he was preparing to return to the United States, he asked Neem Karoli Baba what teaching he should take home with him. The sage told him to simply keep asking the question "Who am I?" as he went about his daily activities. Zen masters also use this question as a koan, giving it to students to contemplate.

So, *who am I?*

Am I my body?

No. If I were my body, it would obey the command not to be sick.

Am I my mind?

No. If I were my mind, it would obey the command not to ever feel down or depressed.

Who am I?

In the epigraph that heads this chapter, Joanna Macy answers the question like this: "I am a flow-through of matter, energy, and information." This may not be your answer, but keeping the question in the mind helps break down the sense of a solid, permanent self that leads to fixed (and limiting) identities such as "I am a sick person" or "I am a caregiver for a sick person." Shedding these fixed identities opens possibilities for seeing the world with new eyes.

The answer to "Who am I?" remains a mystery to me—and I'm content with that. Mysteries are compelling and intriguing and, in this case, also quite liberating.

Sky-Gazing Practice

To help me experience no-self, I use a practice called "sky-gazing" from the Dzogchen tradition of Tibetan Buddhism. I lie down in my backyard, look up at the sky, and relax my gaze. After a while, the experience takes on an openness and a spaciousness. All notions of a separate self—in body or in mind—dissolve. There may be a sound or a sensation of a breeze going by or a thought arising, but it's simply energy, flowing through. Although this spaciousness may last only a few seconds, in those seconds, there's no Toni Bernhard.

Even when the illusion of Toni Bernhard reemerges as a solid, separate entity (as it always does!), those few seconds without it are so liberating that a serene glow stays with me for a while. Gradually the glow fades and identities start piling on: former dean and law professor, wife, mother, dog owner, sick person. But I can always sky-gaze again.

I use a variation of sky-gazing while lying in bed, especially at night when I'm unable to sleep due to pain or other symptoms. I close my eyes and consciously switch my focus away from awareness of unpleasant bodily sensations by letting my pupils

44   *Pain Is Part of Life*

roll upward toward the top of my head. This signals that I've made a shift in consciousness that's the equivalent of sky-gazing. Soon identities start peeling away, including the identity "sick person." The body is experienced as pulsating matter, teeming with energy. The mind is experienced as a conduit for information that flows in and flows out.

"No self, no problem," a popular Buddhist saying goes. And everything is okay just as it is—sickness and all.

Finding Peace and Joy

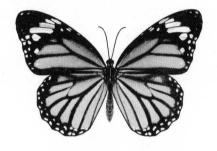

6

Finding Joy in the Life You Can No Longer Lead

We should find perfect existence through imperfect existence.
—SHUNRYU SUZUKI

AS WITH MANY oral traditions that transmit their spiritual teachings from generation to generation by word of mouth, the Buddha's teachings were often passed down in lists—like the Four Noble Truths and the Eightfold Path, which many people have heard of even though they've never studied Buddhism. Lists work because they make the teachings easier to commit to memory. Nevertheless, Buddhists like to joke about both the staggering number of lists and how so many concepts appear on multiple lists.

No matter which list we use to enter the teachings, it won't be long before we reach the Buddha's core teaching: the fact of mental suffering in our lives and the practices that can lead to the end of that suffering.

For me, the sweetest list is what the Buddha called the *brahma viharas,* often translated as the four "sublime states." I love the dictionary definition of *sublime*: "so awe-inspiringly beautiful as

49

to seem heavenly." Simply put, these are mental states we would be wise to cultivate because they are the dwelling place of a mind that is awake and free. Indeed, in Pali, *vihara* means "dwelling place."

The four sublime states are the following:

Metta—kindness; treating ourselves and others with openhearted warmth and friendliness
Karuna—compassion; reaching out to help alleviate suffering in others as well as ourselves
Mudita—empathetic joy; feeling joyful when others are happy
Upekkha—equanimity; being at peace no matter what our circumstances

Neem Karoli Baba often told his disciples, "Don't throw anyone out of your heart"—and "anyone" would, of course, include ourselves. This one powerful sentence encompasses all four sublime states, and I would only temper his words by invoking the same intention as the Zen teacher Robert Aitken did whenever he began a recitation of the Buddhist precepts: "I undertake the practice of . . ." I like this because words such as *don't* or *always* can set us up for failure. I won't always succeed in my efforts to cultivate the four sublime states, but I vow to undertake the practice of cultivating them—the practice of not throwing anyone out of my heart.

Cultivating empathetic joy (the subject of this chapter; the next three chapters will cover the other sublime states) has been central to coming to terms with the life I can no longer lead. Without the ability to share others' joy—*even just a little*—I'd be steeped in envy. Because our activities are so limited, it's hard for the chronically ill not to feel overwhelmed by envy for those who are fortunate enough to be able to keep doing the things they always have. Many of us must stay at home, unable to join family and friends when they go to a movie, or take a bike ride, or go on vacation, or attend a wedding or other major life event.

Even those who are not housebound have to pace themselves carefully and cannot always spontaneously visit or go out for a meal with family and friends. These limitations often apply to caregivers, too, because they must frequently forgo cherished activities either because their loved ones need care or because the activities aren't enjoyable to engage in alone. Tony finds it hard to enjoy weddings and the like without having me there to share the experience with him and to talk together about it afterward.

So it's not surprising that envy arises easily in the life of the chronically ill and their caregivers. It can be so overpowering that it feels as if it's eating us alive—and it has sometimes been like that for me. When envy is strong, it drives away any chance of feeling peaceful and serene. In addition, the emotional stress brought on by envy exacerbates our physical symptoms. The latter is not surprising; Buddhism understands an emotion to be a thought plus a physical reaction to that thought.

Thankfully, empathetic joy can be a powerful antidote to the emotional pain of envy. After becoming ill, it took me a long time to be able to evoke this sublime state easily. At first, feeling joyful just because others were happy was a sheer act of will. I'd learn that people I knew were going to the Mendocino coast, which used to be a favorite haunt for Tony and me, and envy would rear its ugly head. I'd think of this practice and try to feel happy about it, silently saying, "It's so nice they'll be seeing the ocean," but I'd be saying it through gritted teeth. It felt like fake joy. I stuck with the practice, though, and slowly, slowly, slowly fake joy began to turn into genuine joy.

Here's a crucial point, and it doesn't only apply to empathetic joy—it applies to all four sublime states. Their cultivation is not to be looked upon as a pass/fail test. For example, with empathetic joy, if you feel even a bit of joy in the midst of envy, you've succeeded and can cultivate that seed, knowing that you're heading in the right direction.

That's why sticking with a practice even though it might feel artificial or fake still allows that practice to enter your heart, your mind, and your body. This begins to change your conditioned response. With empathetic joy, as your ability to share others' joy grows stronger, you'll feel better yourself. For me, this is the magic of practicing this sublime state: feeling joy for others feels good because when you feel others' joy, that feeling resonates in you, giving rise to feeling joyful yourself.

It took time and patience with this practice for me to feel joyful along with others. At first, when Tony would call from his cell phone while he and our granddaughter Malia were off on an adventure in Los Angeles—at the California Science Center, the Santa Monica Pier, the La Brea Tar Pits—envy would arise in my mind and take hold of me like the tar in those pits. I *hated* not being there. I hated not being able to fulfill the dream I'd had of being an active grandparent, showing Malia all around the city of my birth.

I vividly remember one incident in particular when I not only found myself feeling envious of one of Tony's trips to see Malia, but I was also downright resentful. Envy arises when we want what others have or can do. Resentment is also present if we believe we're not getting it because of some perceived injustice in the world.

Tony had bought tickets for the two of them to go to *Fiddler on the Roof* while he was visiting in Los Angeles. This musical is special to me because it's the story of how my father's family immigrated from modern-day Ukraine to the United States in the early 1900s; they left because of the pogroms against Jews. *Fiddler on the Roof* was *my* story, and I wanted to be the one to take Malia to see it. As a result, instead of feeling happy about their plans, I felt envy and resentment—I felt like the victim of some terrible injustice because I was too sick to travel. "It's not fair!" I protested to myself.

With effort, I was able to turn my misery around. I started by evoking self-compassion for how hard it was not to be able to take Malia to *Fiddler*. Being kind to myself in this way enabled me to drop the painful stories I was spinning about how unfair life can be. It also made it easier to look at their plans through their eyes and reflect on how they wouldn't want their evening at *Fiddler* to make me unhappy.

Then I turned my attention to feeling empathetic joy. Again, at first I had to pretend, but that's okay. It didn't take long for that pretending to turn into genuine joy as I felt happy just knowing that Malia was going to see a musical that's such an important part of my life. And then something special happened. The joy I was feeling made me feel so connected to them that it felt as if I were part of the evening, too—as if the two of them were there for all three of us.

Cultivating the sublime state of empathetic joy may be an ongoing challenge but, for me, it's been a great gift from the Buddha. To paraphrase Shunryu Suzuki's words at the beginning of this chapter: empathetic joy has allowed me to find perfect existence, even though my heath is far from perfect.

7

Soothing the Body, Mind, and Heart

May the gentle breeze and the calm sea
protect your loved ones and friends on their journey.
—"SOAVE SIA IL VENTO"
FROM MOZART'S *COSÌ FAN TUTTE*

METTA, KINDNESS, is the act of treating ourselves and others with openhearted friendliness. We're unlikely to be able to love all the people who pass through our lives, but we can be kind and friendly and wish that no harm comes to them. This practice differs from compassion in that, traditionally, the latter is directed toward those who are suffering. By contrast, metta is directed toward everybody, from the mail carrier, to loved ones, to those you'd rather not see at all (including on your TV screen).

In traditional metta practice, you settle on a set of phrases and then recite them silently, over and over. The phrases can be directed to yourself, to others as a whole, or to particular people. These are the phrases I settled on in the early 1990s:

May I be peaceful.
May I have ease of well-being
May I reach the end of suffering . . .
And be free.

There's no magic to these four phrases. The cadence and meaning just work for me. "Ease of well-being" is a phrase I first heard from the Buddhist teacher Sharon Salzberg. I like it because it suggests that we greet each moment of everyday life with care and kindness. It's as if I'm saying, "May I have ease of well-being as I shower . . . as I eat this meal . . . as I lie down to nap . . . and even as I experience sickness, fatigue, and pain." Other possible phrases: "May I be happy. May my mind be healed. May I make friends with my body. May I dwell in peace."

After taking some time to try out different phrases, it's best to settle on one set. The act of listening to and contemplating the meaning of the phrases as you repeat them, over time, softens and soothes the body, mind, and heart. In fact, now I need only silently say, "May I be peaceful," and it sets off a relaxation response in my mind and body. They know what's coming next! Sometimes I remove myself as the subject altogether and just lie in bed, repeating, "Peaceful, ease of well-being, end of suffering, free."

The phrase "end of suffering" should be familiar from the discussion of the Four Noble Truths in chapter 3. When my health didn't return, I lay in bed repeating my chosen metta phrases. One day when I got to "May I reach the end of suffering," I became aware that I was wishing I'd stop feeling sick—that the physical discomfort would *go away*, that I would *stop being sick*. Of course, wishing for something over which I had no control only brought more suffering.

It was then that I realized that most of my suffering came not from the physical discomfort of the illness but from my mind reacting to it with thoughts such as "I don't want to be sick," "I hate this physical discomfort," "What if I can never return to work?" A shift occurred, and the end of suffering I wished for became the end of suffering *in the mind*. In fact, I could add "in the mind" to the end of each of my four chosen phrases, whether I'm directing them at myself or at others.

Although I've settled on the above set of phrases for my basic metta practice, I use other words at times. For example, while on the July 2001 retreat I wrote about earlier, I dragged myself to a talk given by Kamala Masters because, sick though I was, I loved being in her calm and serene presence. That evening she closed her talk by directing this phrase to us: "Whether sick or well, may your body be a vehicle for liberation." That got my attention! I didn't replace one of my four phrases with this one, but while lying in bed I still sometimes silently repeat, "Sick though it is, may this body be a vehicle for liberation."

Traditionally, metta phrases are directed toward different groups of people. You start with yourself and then move progressively from those for whom it is easiest for you to evoke feelings of kindness and friendliness to those who are the hardest.

First, direct the phrases at yourself. This opens your heart to the practice. It's difficult to feel kind toward others if you're not feeling kind toward yourself. If you feel resistance at first, that's okay. Many of us have been conditioned to be our own harshest critics, making it hard for us to speak kindly to ourselves. If this is true for you, I suggest you think of that cliché, "This is the first day of the rest of your life," and imagine a blank slate in your mind. Begin to fill that slate with thoughts of kindness, benevolence, and friendliness toward yourself. Repeat your phrases even if they don't feel genuine at first. They will work their magic anyway, transforming your heart and mind.

After taking some time to direct the phrases at yourself, call to mind someone for whom you feel deep gratitude and address the phrases to this person. Then move to a person you love but toward whom you might also have some conflicting feelings (such as a close friend or loved one). Then pick a person you don't have an opinion about one way or another (such as a cashier at the supermarket).

Finally, address your phrases to a person whose name alone gives rise to anger, judgment, and other thoughts and emotions that are a source of suffering for you. This last category is called "the difficult person" and is one of the most powerful aspects of this practice. It can be hard to direct thoughts of kindness toward a person who is a source of difficulty for you. He or she could be a family member, a doctor who doesn't take your illness seriously, or even a public figure. Wishing for a person who is a thorn in your side to be peaceful and to be free from suffering may be a challenge, but it's an antidote for anger and ill will, which turns this practice into a liberating one.

For the difficult person, I usually pick a politician—someone with whom I vehemently disagree—to be the object of my kind and friendly thoughts. First, recognizing that my reaction to this person is a source of suffering *for me*, I begin by directing kind thoughts toward myself: "May I be free from the suffering that my aversion to this person gives rise to." Then I turn my attention to the person: "May you be peaceful. May you have ease of well-being. May you reach the end of suffering . . . and be free."

At first the phrases feel artificial and fake. But as I've trained myself to do, I persist. Soon, not only do the phrases become genuine but I also begin to see qualities in the person that I share. For instance, perhaps we both have families we love. Perhaps the person clings to his or her political views as tenaciously as I cling to mine—a shared source of suffering for us!

After a time, it feels as if a poison has been extracted from my body, mind, and heart. Practicing this sublime state is an antidote for hatred and ill will toward others. The politician in question probably still won't get my vote, but evoking feelings of kindness toward him or her frees me from the anger and ill will that are the sources of mental suffering and that often intensify my physical symptoms as well.

I hope you'll work on treating others as well as yourself with kindness and openhearted friendliness. It can soothe a body that's sick or in pain, and offers peace to a troubled mind or a hardened heart.

8

Using Compassion to Alleviate Your Suffering

When the heart at last acknowledges how much pain
there is in the mind, it turns like a mother
toward a frightened child.
—STEPHEN LEVINE

COMPASSION, the third sublime state, is described in Buddhism as the quivering of the heart in response to the recognition of suffering. Once we recognize the presence of suffering in ourselves and others, our practice is to look for ways to help alleviate it. In this chapter, I'm going to focus on cultivating compassion for ourselves because, for many of us, this is harder than cultivating compassion for others.

The four sublime states are not mutually exclusive; I may call upon more than one of them at a time to help me through a difficulty. Recall the story about how I cultivate empathetic joy when Tony and my granddaughter Malia call while they're out and about in Los Angeles. Sometimes that call comes on a day when I'm feeling particularly sick or mentally down because of my limitations. Although I seldom feel envy when they tell me what they're doing, it may be too difficult for me to feel joyful. When this happens, I evoke compassion for the emotional pain I'm experiencing at not being able to join them. This never fails to ease my suffering.

Before I became chronically ill, two teachers helped me "recondition" my mind so that compassion became a natural response to my own suffering. The first teacher was Thich Nhat Hanh. In his book *The Diamond That Cuts through Illusion*, he describes how the body responds naturally—without thought—to its own pain: "When our left hand is injured, our right hand takes care of it right away. It doesn't stop to say, 'I am taking care of you. You are benefiting from my compassion.'"

Indeed, when I fell and broke my ankle, before any thoughts about it arose in my mind, my hands had already reached out to care for the pain. With practice, we can condition the mind to respond compassionately to our pain and suffering, just as our hands do.

The second teacher who helped me learn to cultivate compassion for myself was Mary Grace Orr. On a Spirit Rock retreat in the late 1990s, she told a story that had a profound effect on me. She was describing a harried day in which she had too much to do and too little time in which to do it. (Sound familiar?) At one point, while in her car, she realized she was talking to herself in a way she would never talk to others. I don't remember her exact words, but they immediately resonated with me because of their similarity to the way I used to talk to myself:

"How stupid of me to take this route; it's always full of traffic."

"I'm so dumb, I forgot to bring my notebook."

"You clumsy idiot—you dropped your drink again."

Would I ever call Tony "dumb" or "stupid" or an "idiot"? No! And what's more, if I ever heard someone talking like this to someone I cared about—or even to a stranger—I would at least feel the impulse to intervene. Mary's story was an eye-opener for me. From then on, when I'd catch myself using that language, I'd stop and reflect on how I'd never talk to others that way. After a few months, I had "reconditioned" my mind to treat my own difficulties with compassion.

Then I got sick and that reconditioning unraveled.

I blamed myself for not recovering from the initial viral infection—as if not regaining my health was my fault: a failure of will, somehow, or a deficit of character. This is a common reaction for people to have toward their illness. It's not surprising, given that our culture tends to treat chronic illness as some kind of personal failure on the part of the afflicted—a bias that's often implicit or unconscious but is nonetheless palpable. I was helped by Tony and by Spirit Rock teacher Sylvia Boorstein, who kept reminding me that this illness was just this illness, not a personal failing on my part. In the end, it took an intense moment of physical and mental suffering for me to finally reach out to myself with compassion.

It happened on Thanksgiving. At that time I'd been sick for a year and a half, but I was still not willing to accept that I could no longer travel to family events. So I agreed to go to Escondido where, for years, my daughter-in-law's parents, Bob and Jacqueline Lawhorn, hosted us for Thanksgiving. I planned the trip to accommodate my illness. Tony would drive down from Davis; I would get a ride to the airport and take a plane from Sacramento, which would shorten my travel time; and I'd only stay for two days.

The moment Tony picked me up at the San Diego airport and we began the forty-five-minute drive to Escondido, I knew the trip had been a mistake. We checked into our hotel and drove to the Lawhorns' house. After ten minutes of visiting, I felt so sick that the room began to spin and I couldn't focus on people. I told

Jacqueline that I needed to lie down. Except for sleeping at the hotel at night, I spent that day and the next on the Lawhorns' bed. I felt no compassion for myself. I was ashamed of being sick and I blamed myself for everything my mind could come up with: undertaking the trip in the first place; taking over the Lawhorns' bedroom (which they graciously gave me, of course); not visiting with family and friends; ruining Tony's Thanksgiving. The list was long because, as Jack Kornfield likes to say, "The mind has no shame."

On Friday, Tony dropped me off at the San Diego airport. The flight was delayed two hours. I propped myself up in the chairs near the gate as best I could. I'd arranged for the Davis Airporter, a minivan service, to pick me up at the Sacramento airport. I walked outside the terminal to find that Sacramento was socked in with tule fog—a cold, wet fog that descends on the Central Valley in winter. The van wasn't there yet, so I sat on my suitcase in the fog. Since getting sick, this was the closest I'd come to collapsing on the ground. When the van pulled up about fifteen minutes later, the driver told me that he had to wait for two other planes to arrive before he could drive to Davis. I got in the van and lay down on the seat to wait. It was cold and damp. Ten minutes. Fifteen minutes. Twenty minutes. My physical suffering was matched only by my mental suffering in the form of the hatred and blame I was directing at myself.

Then suddenly, unexpectedly, there was a turning of the mind, and my heart opened. Maybe, on a subconscious level, I was recalling Mary Grace Orr's story, and I knew I'd never treat another person the way I was treating myself. Maybe I was finally ready to receive Tony and Sylvia's compassionate reminder that this illness was not a personal failing on my part. I'm not sure what caused this change of heart and mind, but I got out of the van, explained to the driver that I was sick, and asked if he could

64   *Finding Peace and Joy*

please call the dispatcher and get permission to take me to Davis. He called, got permission immediately, and drove me home. That experience marked the beginning of my ability to treat this illness with compassion.

One of my favorite compassion practices is *tonglen*, which comes from the Tibetan Buddhist tradition. Chapter 11 will explore that practice in detail. Here I'm going to offer five other practices I use to cultivate compassion for myself.

Disidentify from Your Inner Critic

Most of us have been conditioned from childhood to be our own harshest critics. That inner judge can shadow us, scrutinizing our every move and giving us negative feedback that makes us feel bad about ourselves. When I first became sick, the inner critic was *in charge.* For several years I've been working to turn that inner critic into an inner ally who will refuse to disparage me, just as I refuse to disparage those I care about. Taming the inner critic is truly an act of self-compassion.

The practice that has been most helpful is called *disidentifying*— that is, not treating the inner critic voice as an authentic, fixed feature of yourself. Disidentifying in this way can take several forms. For instance, you can give the critic a name: "Oh, it's Ms. Nag again." Doing this keeps you from identifying with the voice as an immutable part of your personality.

Another effective disidentifying technique is to imagine that the inner critic is a voice on a stage and you're in the audience, watching the performance. Here's what I do: When I become aware that the inner critic has shown up, I put it on stage and imagine myself in the balcony of a theater, listening to it go on and on about how Toni shouldn't have gotten sick and how she shouldn't have gotten breast cancer. As a member of the audience, I hear the absurdity of that voice's criticisms—does it think this Toni has the ability to control everything that happens in her life, including the ability to make sure that all her experiences are pleasant ones? When I disidentify with that voice by putting it on a stage, I find myself thinking, "Someone should show that critical voice the Buddha's list from the first noble truth!"

Then I (as an audience member) consider what would make for better "onstage" viewing and listening. The answer is easy: a focus on the positives in Toni's life, despite her health problems. For starters, she has a roof over her head, a loving partner, and a cuddly dog. There's a lot of lovely stuff that could be showcased on that stage instead of incessant nagging criticism.

Disidentifying from the inner critic brings into sharp focus the impossible standards we often hold ourselves to. All of us do this to some extent—we cling to an idea of how we think we *should* be—but this just encourages the inner critic to pay a visit. Then not only is it impossible for us to feel compassion for our mental or physical suffering, but we're also unable to tap into any joy that's present for us right now.

I hope you'll try one of these disidentifying techniques the next time your inner critic shows up. You'll recognize that the critic is present because you'll hear the words *should* and *shouldn't*, and you'll realize that you're directing blame at yourself. That's the signal to disidentify from that negative inner voice, either by giving it a name that's not associated with you or by imagining it's on a stage and you're a neutral third party in the balcony being forced to listen to its negative chatter.

66   *Finding Peace and Joy*

Craft Phrases That Directly Address Your Suffering

I'm always coming across articles that tell me to treat myself with compassion, but they rarely explain how to go about it. Here's what I've discovered about turning self-compassion into a living, breathing practice: Rather than using nonspecific phrases such as "May I be free from suffering," choose a set of words that speak directly to the specific circumstances that are making you sad, disappointed, or dispirited. Then repeat the phrases to yourself. I usually do this silently, but you could whisper or even talk out loud if the environment is appropriate for that.

If speaking to yourself seems odd, reflect on how your inner critic doesn't have any trouble speaking words of criticism to you. If you can talk to yourself in harsh and self-judgmental ways, there's no reason not to talk to yourself in soothing, gentle, self-compassionate ways instead. If it feels fake at first, that's okay. You're learning a new skill and it takes time. The Buddha said that the mind is as flexible as the balsam tree, so we can change old habits and develop new, more wholesome ones. With practice, cultivating self-compassion can become a lifelong habit, one you can depend on to restore your spirits. As a bonus, when you speak this way to yourself, the inner critic doesn't stand a chance!

I relied on this practice during the months when I had to wait for test results relating to breast cancer. And I've continued to use the practice to help me cope with the possibility that the cancer might recur. It turns out that with cancer, there's a lot of waiting. First I had to wait for test results that led to the need for a biopsy. Then I had to wait for the results of the biopsy. Then for the results of an MRI. That led to a lumpectomy, and then I had to wait more than two weeks for the results of pathology tests on my lymph nodes and on tissue samples from the surgery (thankfully, both were negative). And even after discussing the results of the pathology tests with my surgical oncologist, I had to wait to hear how the next specialists in line (the radiology oncologist and the medical oncologist) interpreted the results so they could recommend a course of postsurgical treatment. And, of course, now there's "chronic waiting" to see if the cancer returns.

While waiting for test results, when I felt overwhelmed by the desire to have all the answers immediately, I spoke silently or softly to myself in a kind voice: "It's so hard to want the results *right now* but not have control over when they'll be available." When I was struggling to get to sleep one night because of anxiety over a crucial consult the next day, I said to myself, "Rest peacefully, sweet body; rest peacefully, sweet mind." And, regarding a recurrence, I sometimes say, "It's really tough to feel so uncertain about the future of my health."

Speaking to myself in this way helps me acknowledge and accept without bitterness the truth of the human condition—that there's a lot about life that we don't control and that not all our experiences will be pleasant. Finally, it heightens my awareness of others who are in the same situation, and this helps me feel less alone.

I suggest you try this practice by focusing on whatever specific challenges and disappointments you're facing. We know from the first and second noble truths that dukkha can be traced to our Want/Don't-Want Mind, so think about something you want but aren't getting or something you're getting but don't want. Then craft some phrases that directly address this suffering.

You might use phrases such as "It's hard to be in too much pain to go out with friends" or "I'm sad that I had to miss the party." Be careful that your words aren't a backdoor way to blame yourself for your limitations: "I'm so disappointed that I have to let my friends and family down again." To see if your words are

68   *Finding Peace and Joy*

genuinely intended to alleviate your suffering, ask if these are words you'd use to comfort a loved one who shared his or her suffering with you.

Speaking directly to the source of your suffering can also become a powerful forgiveness practice. On a day when I'm mentally low due to feeling particularly sick or in pain, I might repeat to myself, "Take care, sweet body, working so hard to support me." When I repeat a phrase with that sentiment, I'm also forgiving myself for becoming chronically ill. This struggle with my health is not my body's fault; it's doing the best it can to support me.

Finally, sometimes when I speak compassionate phrases to myself, I stroke one arm with the hand of the other—a practice I learned from Thich Nhat Hanh in his *Diamond That Cuts through Illusion*. This has brought me to tears sometimes, but tears of compassion are healing tears.

Take the Initiative to Connect with Others

The idea for this next self-compassion practice came from a talk on generosity given by Sharon Salzberg at a Spirit Rock retreat. She suggested that as soon as a thought arises to be generous (call a friend in need, give something away simply because someone admires it), we should resolve to follow through on that generous impulse even though we may subsequently try to talk ourselves out of it with thoughts such as "I'm too busy to call" or "On second thought, I want that item I was going to give away." I had used this practice for many years. Not only did it benefit others, but I also found it highly amusing to reflect on the rationalizations I could come up with for talking myself out of that initial impulse to be generous: "Hmm, if I'm ever invited to the White House, I might want to wear that scarf . . ."

After that transformative experience at Thanksgiving, I looked for ways to alleviate the suffering that accompanied my illness. One day, I stumbled upon a way to change Sharon's generosity practice into a compassion practice for myself. Although the practices are quite different, I must give Sharon credit because I wouldn't have thought of mine had it not been for the wisdom of hers.

The practices are different because, instead of following through on an initial impulse to be generous, I force myself, in this compassion practice, to do the reverse of my initial impulse. Here's an example of how it works. If my two children haven't been in touch for a while, as soon as the thought arises, "Why don't they contact me?" I immediately contact *them*. So instead of allowing that thought, "Why don't they contact me?" to spin out into the many absurd storylines it could take ("They'd like me better if I weren't sick"; "I bore them"), I "cut off the mind road" (to use a Zen saying we'll encounter again in chapter 15) and force myself to contact them. It's as if my "penalty" for thinking that they should contact *me* is that I have to contact *them*!

The results are always uplifting and never fail to alleviate the suffering brought about by the proliferation of thoughts that weren't true. When I contact my children, we talk about what they've been up to. We talk about my grandchildren. We share common experiences—maybe a movie or a sporting event on TV we've both seen. They may seek my advice. It always becomes clear as we're talking that they've been thinking about me. Sometimes it turns out they've been busy. (Didn't I want them to be independent as adults and to live full lives? Yes!) Sometimes it turns out they've been sick themselves.

The principal feature that Sharon's practice and my practice share is how, unless we remain vigilant by cultivating awareness—often called "mindfulness"—the mind can talk us into or out of just about anything, no matter how counterproductive or harmful the consequences.

Here's another example of how I've used this practice. My friend Dawn tries to visit me for a short time every week. She lives over an hour away but comes to Davis often. One time, Tony was at a meditation retreat. He'd left on a Friday. Dawn was going to visit on Tuesday. But two days after Tony left, I lost the benefit I'd been experiencing from a new treatment and had a big setback in my condition. I had to cancel our visit. She said she could visit on Wednesday instead, but I had to cancel that, too. I was just too sick.

Come Friday night, I suddenly felt resentful that, knowing I wasn't doing well, Dawn hadn't checked in with me. As soon as that resentful thought arose, the "penalty" kicked in, meaning I had to cut off the negative thoughts that were about to proliferate and, instead, immediately contact her. I forced myself to pick up my laptop and send her an email. I wrote a short paragraph about my rough week and then asked how she and her family were doing. She wrote back right away. Her email started with this sentence: "I had been thinking about you, but I think I was afraid to ask you how you were doing. I won't do that again."

Here I'd been judging her negatively only to find out that not only had she been thinking about me but she also had a reason for not getting in touch; sometimes it's just too hard for people to hear how poorly a friend is doing. In addition, it turned out she'd had a particularly busy week—hosting visitors from out of town, taking care of two of her grandchildren, and negotiating the purchase of some property that was located a few hours from where she lived. A full plate indeed. Once again, the storyline I'd spun regarding someone else's motives failed to reflect what was really going on.

Practicing compassion is the act of reaching out to ourselves and to others to help alleviate suffering. By using the practice I just described, instead of allowing stressful thoughts about family and friends to proliferate and then fester, I consciously shift my mental state and take action. That action never fails to alleviate my suffering and, as a bonus, gives me a big lift.

Cultivate Patient Endurance

The fourth way I cultivate compassion for myself is to practice *khanti*, usually translated as "patience." (Warning: it's part of another Buddhist list!) Khanti is one of the ten "practices of perfection": ten qualities that a buddha, or enlightened one, has perfected. Two of the four sublime states—kindness and equanimity—are also on this list. The other seven are generosity, moral conduct, renunciation, wisdom, energy, truthfulness, and determination. In *Being Nobody, Going Nowhere*, Ayya Khema says of the ten perfections, "We have their seed in us. If that were not so, we would be cultivating barren ground."

Ayya Khema was a native German Jew who, after escaping the Nazis, became a Theravada Buddhist nun in Sri Lanka. At a retreat in Northern California in 1996, she told us that she prefers the words *patient endurance* to *patience* alone and that maintaining patient endurance is the most difficult part of Buddhist practice. Ayya Khema's rendering transforms what could be seen as a passive state of mind ("just be patient") into an active practice. *Patient endurance* suggests that, in addition to being patient (that is, serene and uncomplaining), we actively "endure"; we survive difficulties, we face hardship without giving up.

I include patient endurance on my list of compassion practices because it can help alleviate our suffering as we face the many difficulties that result from being chronically ill. Cultivating patient endurance can help caregivers, too, because they often find themselves in the role of "patient advocate" for their loved one.

One recurring challenge is the uncommon number of hours spent navigating the health-care system. I've found that when dealing with the health-care system, if I don't "endure" I often don't get decent service. At the same time, if I'm not "patient" the frustration stemming from the interaction exacerbates my symptoms. Indeed, patience is a strong antidote to anger—a state of mind that is the source of so much suffering.

One of the most trying odysseys with my health-care provider involved a prescription drug recommended to me by an expert in ME/CFS at Harvard. Of all things, it's produced from pig's liver. *In vitro*, it has proven to have antiviral qualities and is approved by the FDA to treat some skin conditions. First, I had to get my doctor to prescribe the drug. Not surprisingly, he was reluctant when I raised it as a possible treatment. This would be an off-label use of a drug so esoteric that it didn't even appear in his prescription drug manuals. Plus, I'd have to learn to inject myself at home. It took about a month for him to read over the research materials I'd brought him and do his own investigation, but in the end he agreed.

With that taken care of, I approached my insurance company. They had no obligation to approve this off-label use of the drug, but I thought it was worth a try because it was so expensive. After three lengthy phone calls, I succeeded in getting approval for a three-month trial period. It was February. The representative said that the three-month trial would expire on May 15. Even though these lengthy phone calls were exhausting, I was happy with this result. Little did I know the difficulties were just beginning.

The drug was imported from New Zealand and only one pharmacy in the United States was authorized to dispense it. Despite this, my insurance company insisted I use the pharmacy that they contracted with to dispense injectable drugs. I tried over and over to explain to the representative that the pharmacy she was trying to send me to would not have access to the drug. She would not listen. At times during this conversation, I could feel impatience beginning to arise. I wanted to get pushy with her, but I knew it wouldn't change her position and would only intensify my symptoms. As it was, I was exhausted from the interaction. "Patience," I silently repeated to myself. "Patiently endure."

Like a soldier on a mission she knows cannot be accomplished, I called the pharmacy she said I had to use. To my surprise, I was told, "No problem. We'll dispense it." I hung up, feeling a bit sheepish. But there was no time for reflection because I had a third call to make—to my doctor to tell him to fax the prescription to this particular pharmacy. He did so. Mission accomplished?

Oh, no.

The next day, a woman from the pharmacy called to tell me what I already knew. I must use the pharmacy with the sole dispensing rights for the drug. And she said it was *my* responsibility to call my insurance company and inform them. I felt as if I were on a Möbius strip, taking action after action but always winding up back where I started.

I took a deep breath and began again. I was already physically and mentally exhausted from spending so much time on the phone. I didn't want to double my misery by allowing impatience to take hold. So with patient endurance as my protector, I called my insurance company and succeeded in getting the representative to phone the company's contracting pharmacy and get confirmation that it could not dispense the medication. A couple of phone calls later and I thought everything was in place. My doctor would refax the prescription to the pharmacy with the sole dispensing rights. All I had to do was wait a few hours and then call the pharmacy to arrange for shipment.

In excitement, I made the call. They were out of the drug. It had been shipped from New Zealand but was stuck in Australian customs. For the next three months, I called this pharmacy once a week. Each time I was given a new ETA. By the time the medication arrived in the States, it was after May 15 and so the three-month trial period approved by my health insurance company had expired. Time for yet another phone call. The insurance representative told me there was no provision for an extension of an approved trial period, so I'd have to start all over if I wanted them to reconsider approving the drug. Möbius strip. Help! Patience needed!

In the end, I obtained this much sought-after and hard-won medication—and it did nothing whatsoever to improve my condition. But the moral of this tale is that it might have helped (it has helped others) and so, looking back, it was the continual cultivation of patient endurance that gave me the opportunity to try the treatment. *Patience* enabled me to pursue getting the medication while keeping the exacerbation of my symptoms to a minimum. *Endurance* enabled me to make that "one more phone call" that eventually got me the result I was after.

Sometimes being chronically ill feels like a full-time job. While I perform this work, I keep patient endurance at my side. It's a self-compassion practice because it helps keep frustration and anger from arising—two states of mind that are always waiting in the wings when I have to navigate the health-care system.

Open Your Heart to Your Suffering

The fifth way I cultivate compassion for myself is to consciously work on opening my heart to the intense emotions—and emotional swings—that accompany chronic illness. This practice began quite unexpectedly after my daughter's family had come up from Los Angeles for Labor Day weekend. I was three months into a new treatment and was feeling optimistic about its prospects. Tony and I thought this might be the one, and indeed, I'd been able to spend more time than usual that weekend visiting with everyone. But the morning after they left, I awoke feeling like my old sick self.

As I lay in bed that day I began to fear that this treatment, like the others, was going to be a disappointment. The fear grew more and more intense, so I began to follow an instruction I learned early on in mindfulness practice: labeling thoughts and emotions. "Fear, fear—this is fear," I silently repeated. Sometimes it's difficult to label stressful mental states without falling prey to aversion, as in, "Fear; this is fear. It's time to go away, fear. Get out of here *now*!" I've practiced labeling thoughts and emotions myriad times, both in and out of meditation, but this time something different happened. As I noted "fear . . . fear," instead of passively waiting for it to pass on through, there was a shift in consciousness and I opened to it. Then the thought arose: "My heart is big enough to hold this fear."

And so alongside all the other experiences of my life, I made room for fear. I felt a great spaciousness and expansiveness. Soon I became aware that a gentle smile had appeared on my lips, as if to say, "Ah, yes. My old friend, fear." The seed was sown for a new compassion practice: opening my heart to the full range of emotions that life has in store for me.

At first you may resist these suggestions for treating yourself with compassion. Many of us have to overcome a lifetime of conditioning in which we were taught that looking after our own well-being is selfish. It's not. We are as worthy of our care and compassion as anyone.

Before I learned to cultivate compassion for myself as a chronically ill person, I passively accepted whatever happened. No matter how intense my suffering, I took no action to alleviate it because I blamed myself for being sick. I recall, for example, an appointment I had with an ear, nose, and throat specialist in the fall of 2001 to evaluate a persistent hoarseness that was a feature of the acute phase of the illness. I dragged myself out of bed for Tony to drive us to the clinic only to find that we had to wait three hours to be seen. I tried every position I could think of to turn the waiting-room chair into a reclining piece of furniture. I slumped down on my back; I slumped down on my side. Then I tried to use the chair as a bed, bending my knees to get my feet up on it and laying the middle part of my body over the hard armrest and my head on Tony's lap. The physical pain and discomfort was matched by the mental suffering that arose from blaming myself for being sick and subjecting not just me but also Tony to this misery.

Six years later I was taking an antiviral under the supervision of an infectious disease doctor. On the two-hour drive from Davis to the infectious disease clinic, I could lie down in the back of our van, but the wait at the clinic was always longer than the time it took to get there. At the first appointment, I employed my usual techniques of first trying to turn an upright chair into a recliner and then trying to lie across Tony's lap. It took me weeks to recover from that trip. I dreaded the follow-up appointment.

But at that second visit, having already begun to evoke compassion for myself as someone who is ill, after an hour of waiting I calmly and politely told a staff person that I needed to lie down. To my surprise and relief, after a few minutes, she showed us to an empty room and said I could lie on the examining table until the doctor could see me. When I approached the staff person, I didn't complain but neither was I passive. Instead, I took compassionate action on behalf of myself. I hope you'll start cultivating self-compassion this very minute.

I'd like to close this chapter with a quotation often attributed to the Dalai Lama in which he tells us what can happen if we devote our lives to easing suffering in ourselves and others:

> If you want others to be happy, practice compassion.
> If you want to be happy, practice compassion.

9

Facing the Ups and Downs
of Chronic Illness with Equanimity

Let things take their natural course.
Then your mind will become still in any surroundings,
like a clear forest pool. All kinds of wonderful, rare animals
will come to drink at the pool. . . . You will see many
strange and wonderful things come and go, but you
will be still. This is the happiness of the Buddha.

—AJAHN CHAH

EQUANIMITY is the fourth of the sublime states. The dictionary defines it as "mental calmness and evenness of temper, especially in a difficult situation." That's as good a definition as I've seen for this central Buddhist concept and practice. Dwelling in equanimity, we are able to greet whatever is present in the moment, including unpleasant experiences, with a mind that is at peace. Indeed, some teachers equate this mental state with enlightenment—also known as awakening, liberation, or freedom.

For a chronically ill person, equanimity can be a particularly difficult state of mind to sustain, and so it helps to have both

79

inspirational teachings and practical techniques at hand. I find the challenges fall into three categories:

- maintaining equanimity in the face of the barrage of unhelpful, inaccurate, and often insensitive comments people make about chronic illness (which includes chronic pain and mental illness)
- weathering the unpredictability and uncertainty that accompany chronic illness
- feeling overwhelmed with loss—lost health, lost job, lost friends, lost mobility, lost money

Naturally, these challenges are not entirely exclusive to those who are chronically ill. Nevertheless, chronic illness can generate a particular need for equanimity.

Insensitive and Hurtful Comments

Anyone who is chronically ill—especially if, as in my case, the illness is not visible to others—will have encountered the first challenge many times: how are we to maintain evenness of temper and calm in the face of comments from others that, even if well-intentioned, are so off the mark that we feel misunderstood and often disregarded?

My Internet wanderings have revealed that the chronically ill are subject to remarks from family and friends that are eerily identical in content and reveal a profound ignorance about what it's like to struggle with health problems. Here's a sampling of comments, from Australia to Finland to Switzerland to my own ears in Davis:

- "But you don't look sick."
- "No wonder you feel bad; you never go out."

- "I wish I had time to be sick."
- "Just drink coffee."
- "How come you can't work when you're still able to use your computer?"
- "I'm tired all the time, too."
- "I saw you pulling weeds in your front yard; I'm glad you're healthy again."
- "If you were really that sick, you'd be in the hospital."
- "You can't be that sick if you can write a book."

Do any of those sound familiar?

Having a strong grounding in the reality of no-fixed-self (discussed in chapter 5) helps us to maintain equanimity in the face of these types of comments. In *A Still Forest Pool*, Ajahn Chah offers excellent advice on this point:

> If someone curses us and we have no feelings of self, the incident ends with the spoken words, and we do not suffer. If unpleasant feelings arise, we should let them stop there, realizing that the feelings are not us. . . . If we do not stand up in the line of fire, we do not get shot; if there is no one to receive it, the letter is sent back.

I love that phrase: "If there is no one to receive it, the letter is sent back." This is the essence of no-fixed-self and of equanimity. With a mind that is calm and even-tempered, the insensitive comments of others are just not received. Even the word *insensitive* drops away and words just arise and pass through our consciousness. I wish there had been "no one to receive it" when "just drink coffee" was the sole treatment offered to me by a doctor early in the chronic stage of my illness. I was devastated. It was simply too early in the illness for me to handle the comment with any semblance of equanimity. I sat there "in the line of fire"—and indeed I felt as if I'd been shot. Today I'm more likely to "not be there to receive it," in the sense that I would not take it personally. I'd know that the comment was just a reflection of his lack of skill and sensitivity as a doctor. If I felt strong enough on that day, I would "send the letter back" with some constructive feedback on the inappropriateness of the comment.

Unsolicited health advice is one of the hardest categories of comments that both the chronically ill and their caregivers have to field. Countless times, Tony has told me about having to politely listen to people discourse on treatments that range from off-label use of prescription drugs to moving to a different city to the most bizarre-sounding treatments. I'll never forget the time that one person told me that my body was too acidic and I needed to alkalize it by drinking baking soda and water four times a day. Two days later, another person told me my body was too alkaline and I needed to acidify it by drinking apple cider vinegar four times a day.

The most distressing piece of unsolicited advice I've received showed up in my email inbox in response to an article I'd written about my breast cancer diagnosis. The email read: "I'm sorry to hear you have breast cancer. However, because you're already chronically ill, do not, under any circumstances, continue with radiation. It will destroy your immune system." The email arrived two days after I'd completed a course of radiation.

In my article I'd emphasized that my intention in writing it was to share my experiences in a way that would be helpful to others. I didn't ask for treatment advice, but I received a lot of it, including this email, which only had the effect of making me anxious and worried about a treatment I'd just completed.

These types of comments differ from the "If you're really that sick, you'd be in the hospital" variety because the latter are insensitive and trivialize our condition. By contrast, when people offer treatment advice, they're simply trying to be helpful. Unfortunately, it's frustrating and stressful to be told to stop a treatment that you're committed to or to try something you know won't help. The best way to gracefully "not be there to receive" these well-intentioned comments is to cultivate "wise speech"—the subject of chapter 16—but suffice it to say, the Buddha suggests we speak only when what we have to say is true, kind, and helpful.

Wise speech in the face of these suggestions will often be sparse speech, as in, "Thanks for the suggestion." In the early 1990s, my dear friend Anne was dying of cancer. She told me that almost every visitor arrived with a "cure" in hand, from special teas to amulets she was to wear around her neck. She told me that sometimes she wanted to scream, "I'm in the hands of good doctors, and we're doing everything we can to keep me alive. I don't want or need your advice!" But she didn't say it because she didn't want to hurt people who were being kind enough to visit. When Anne raised this dilemma at a counseling session, her therapist suggested that she say "Thank you" and put the item down. Then, as soon as the person left, shove it under her bed. It turned out to be just the advice she needed.

Unpredictability and Uncertainty in the Lives of the Chronically Ill

The chronically ill face each day not knowing if we'll be able to visit with friends and family, if we can manage a trip outside of the house, if we'll have a bad reaction to a new treatment, if a doctor will be considerate or inconsiderate. We can't even predict which symptoms will hit us hard on a particular day. It's difficult to stay calm and serene in these circumstances—for caregivers, too. Before I introduce four equanimity practices that I find helpful,

I'd like to look more deeply into some of the ways that unpredictability and uncertainty show up in the lives of the chronically ill.

Activities with others. For those of us who were always dependable when it came to keeping commitments, this sudden uncertainty in the face of people's expectations for us to make good on our plans can be a source of great anxiety and stress. Although we never feel fully healthy, we do have days when we function better than others. Unfortunately, we can't predict what days those will be. As a result, we may make plans to have a friend over on a particular day but then have to cancel that morning when we're unable to get out of bed.

Treatments. As I said, I've tried many treatments, some for symptom relief, some as possible cures. My body's response to a treatment is unpredictable. When I've undertaken one as a possible "cure," it's been a challenge to sustain a balanced state of mind that would allow me to accept success or failure with calmness and serenity. At the beginning of the experimental use of an antiviral so powerful I was monitored by three doctors, I told myself, "Maybe it will work, maybe it won't. No expectations; it's just an experiment." But when I experienced considerable improvement after six months, I thought, "This is it! Forget that 'maybe, maybe not' stuff, I'm going to recover!" Then when the positive effects of the antiviral reversed, Tony and I were crestfallen. I felt as if I'd plummeted into a deep abyss.

It was an eye-opening experience. I realized that to live gracefully with this illness, I was going to have to do a better job cultivating the evenness of temper that is at the heart of equanimity. As I write, I can think of nine different major treatment regimens I've undertaken that resulted in initial success, only to be followed by disappointment. (One infectious disease doctor surmises that this might happen because my immune system adjusts to each new treatment, gradually reversing its effects.) Nothing illustrates the value of being able to ride the ups and downs of life with equanimity more than the experience of treatments that initially succeed and then fail.

Doctors. Finally, there's the unpredictability of the outcome of seeing yet another new doctor. For the chronically ill and their caregivers, the medical world is like a club we never asked to join but now find ourselves hanging out at all the time. When I first got sick, I approached each referral to a new specialist with high hopes, only to be let down by almost every one of them. Those with chronic illness—especially a mysterious one—have a name for this: the hot potato treatment. And I wasn't being sent from doctor to doctor because I was a difficult patient. Long before getting sick, I'd mastered the art of being a good patient: be prepared, be deferential, be succinct, don't whine or complain.

I'm not indicting the medical profession; that would be painting with too broad a brush. I'm in a good position to know the harm of doing that, having spent my professional life listening to people tell nasty jokes about lawyers being worse than roadkill. My standard in-person response to that was, "Good thing there were lawyers around to represent those plaintiffs in *Brown v. Board of Education.*" That usually did the trick. And, naturally, I've had positive experiences with doctors. I saw an endocrinologist who was honest with me from the start. She said, "I don't know if what's wrong with you is related to your endocrine system, but I'll do my best to find out." She did indeed do her best and showed great compassion when she was unable to help me. I've been given top-notch care by the oncologists at the UC Davis Comprehensive Cancer Center. And my own primary care doctor is remarkable. He's willing to stick with me even though he can't "fix" me, he's open to my suggestions, and he gives generously of his time. He's never let me down.

That said, here's a taste of encounters with doctors that I'm

Facing the Ups and Downs of Chronic Illness with Equanimity 85

sure will sound familiar to those of us who inhabit the world of the chronically ill:

- A rheumatologist looked me in the eyes and told me he was going to make me well. Tony and I were so excited when we left his office. But when the tests he ordered came back normal, he coldly and bluntly told me, "Go back to your family doctor."
- A neurologist told me at my first appointment that I would be his patient. He regaled Tony and me with his expertise about post-viral syndromes, talking at length about the immune and nervous systems. As we did with the rheumatologist, we left his office exhilarated, given his optimism about what he could do for me. But when we returned for a follow-up appointment, he showed a cursory interest in me, focusing instead on impressing the medical student he had in tow. I was treated as tangential to whatever agenda he had in mind with this student. He spent about ten minutes with us and was gone, offering no help. Tony and I left feeling utterly deflated. I still can't explain why the follow-up visit bore no resemblance to the initial workup.
- An infectious disease doctor asked me to email him ahead of our appointment the results of my own online research into possible treatments. I spent hours researching the web, and then writing and carefully editing an email to him that would be succinct but thorough—at some cost to my health. When he came into the examining room, he acknowledged having received the email but said he hadn't read it. When I politely expressed disappointment, he was miffed and said he'd call me when he'd read it. I never heard from him.

▸ Another infectious disease doctor asked me to make a graph of my day-to-day progress on the antiviral treatment he was monitoring. I painstakingly created a chart based on notes I kept in a daily journal. When I was responding well to the medication, he loved my chart, even calling colleagues into the room to look at it. But when the medication's benefits began to wear off, he wouldn't even look at the chart I had so carefully updated since my last appointment. Even worse, he blamed me for the failure of the antiviral. I wasn't resting enough. I wasn't doing the right kind of exercise. I rested at every opportunity, and exercise? It was an exercise just getting to the appointment. When it was clear his treatment wasn't going to work for me, he dropped me . . . like a hot potato.

Equanimity Practices

Here are four equanimity practices that can help with the particular challenges that come with being chronically ill. I hope you'll give each of them a try.

Whatever happens, it's okay. In the 1990s, when the Thai Forest monk Ajahn Jumnian came for his annual visit to Spirit Rock, I faithfully attended. Bubbling over—as he always was—with joy and laughter, one day he suddenly began discoursing on equanimity. I got out a pen and took these notes:

> When people say, "Ajahn, let's go for a beautiful walk," fine, I'll go. If they don't ask, that's fine, too. I don't expect a walk to be any more satisfying than sitting alone. It could be hot or windy out there. If people bring

me delicious food, great. If they don't, great. I need to diet anyway. If I'm feeling good, that's okay. If I'm sick, that's okay, too. It's a great excuse to lie down.

These few sentences, scribbled on a scrap of paper as Jack Kornfield translated, have become the centerpiece of equanimity practice for me. I rediscovered the notes several years after becoming sick. Reading them with my new circumstance in mind, I understood that the essence of equanimity is accepting life as it comes to us without blaming anything or anyone—including ourselves. I'd been getting despondent when a treatment didn't work and becoming angry when a doctor didn't live up to my expectations. I was trying to control the uncontrollable. Some treatments work. Some don't. Some doctors come through for us. Some don't.

My notes from Ajahn Jumnian's visit and my memory of the joy that emanated from him are still inspiring. Now I cultivate equanimity by saying, "If this medication helps, that will be great. If it doesn't, no blame. It wasn't what my body needed." "If this doctor turns out to be responsive, that will be nice. If he or she doesn't, that's okay. Any given doctor is going to be how he or she is going to be. It's not in my control."

I try to remember Ajahn Jumnian's little gem when I'm faced with the unpredictability of being able to participate in activities or visit with people. Early on in my illness, I bought tickets to the Sacramento Opera's production of *Carmen*. I thought that even if Tony and I could only stay for Act I of the matinee, it would still be a wonderful experience. But on the day of the opera, I was too sick to leave the house. I was resentful and angry that we couldn't go through with the plans I'd so carefully made—including calling to find out how long each act lasted and where the closest disabled parking was. The resentment and anger turned to tears, making it

88   Finding Peace and Joy

harder for Tony. I simply did not have a strong enough equanimity practice to handle the uncertainty and unpredictability that had so unexpectedly become my constant companion in life.

Fast-forward six years. An old family friend was in town and Tony invited him to dinner. I carefully arranged my week so I wouldn't have other commitments in the days leading up to the dinner. This greatly increased the likelihood that I'd be able to join him and Tony for a bit, even though I rarely leave the bedroom after five thirty. But on the evening he came, I was too sick to visit. Had we happened to have scheduled the dinner the night before, I would have been able to socialize for a while.

However, I didn't react the same way I had to the missed opera experience. I didn't lie in the bedroom and cry that night. Instead I recalled Ajahn Jumnian's words and said to myself, "If I could have joined them, that would have been nice. Since I can't, that will be okay, too. I'll listen to music or find a movie on TV. As Ajahn Jumnian said, it's a great excuse to lie down!"

The past few years I've been trying a variation of this practice by consciously starting a sentence with these words: "It's okay if . . ." Doing this helps me stay steady and calm when the everyday challenges of chronic illness begin to throw me off balance. For example, on a day I'm feeling particularly sick or my pain levels are high, I'll say to myself, "It's okay if I feel awful today; that's how chronic illness feels sometimes."

The more I do this, the braver I become with my "It's okay if . . ." formulations. Recently I've been trying this out: "It's okay if I'm chronically ill for the rest of my life." Whoa! The rest of my life? Can that ever be okay? It turns out that, for me, it can. If I'm honest with myself, I might very well be chronically ill for the rest of my life. If that's the case, I know from experience that I feel better emotionally and I'm happier the more I can accept that possibility without resentment and bitterness. And so I've been

Facing the Ups and Downs of Chronic Illness with Equanimity 89

continuing with this particular "It's okay if . . ." practice and, at times, I've truly felt at peace with the possibility that chronic illness is here to stay.

I'm grateful to Ajahn Jumnian for giving us a glimpse that day into how his mind works.

Letting go, even just a little. A second equanimity practice comes from another Thai Forest monk, Ajahn Chah, whom we've heard from before. In his book *A Still Forest Pool*, he offers a statement so powerful that I'd committed it to memory long before getting sick:

> If you let go a little, you will have a little peace. If you let go a lot, you will have a lot of peace. If you let go completely, you will know complete peace and freedom. Your struggles with the world will have come to an end.

I love this teaching because it allows me to take baby steps in the direction of equanimity. I've found that before I can even take that first step and "let go a little," I first have to recognize the suffering that arises from my intense desire for certainty and predictability. Just seeing the suffering in that desire loosens its hold on me, whether it's wanting so badly to be at a family gathering or clinging to the hope for positive results from a medication or desiring for a doctor not to disappoint me. Once I see the suffering in my mind, I can begin to let go a little. As soon as I do that, I get a taste of freedom that motivates me to let go a little more.

I used this practice while waiting for my ankle to be x-rayed. There I was, twenty-four hours after slipping down the two steps, my ankle still throbbing in pain, my knees bruised from crawling around the house, my body aching in fatigue from sitting in a wheelchair way beyond my capacity to be in an upright position.

As thoughts whirled around about whether I could handle this injury on top on my illness, I searched for help in coping with the pain in my body and the suffering in my mind. Help came from Ajahn Chah's teaching on letting go. I thought, "I'm suffering because I don't want this to be happening but, like it or not, it *is* happening, so can I let go even just a little—just a baby step?" I could. And, having done that, I could take another baby step. After a few minutes, I was flooded with equanimity—with the taste of freedom that comes with peaceful acceptance of the unexpected complications that arise in our lives.

Our tendency is, of course, to want our desires to be fulfilled. But if our happiness depends on that, we've set ourselves up for a life of suffering. The strength of our equanimity in the face of not getting our way is the measure of whether we will know the peace and freedom to which Ajahn Chah refers. It's the measure of whether, as he said, our "struggles with the world will have come to an end."

In the previous chapter I described how I spoke compassionately to myself while I was waiting for the many test results associated with breast cancer. During that time, I also relied on Ajahn Chah's equanimity practice. When I found myself overcome with worry and fear, first I'd repeat the compassion phrases I'd come up with, acknowledging how hard it was to wait. Then I'd ask myself if I could let go of the worry and the fear *just a little*, since I had no control over the results of the tests anyway. When I let go just a little, the worry and fear lost their tight grip on me, and I could let go a little more. Repeating these baby steps, I was often able to reach a place of calm acceptance that, like it or not, waiting was the order of the day. When that calm acceptance deserted me, I'd go back and start over, first with the self-compassion phrases and then letting go, even just a little.

This can be a powerful practice. Imagine letting go completely, so that it's okay if you can't go to a family event, a medication doesn't help, or a doctor is disappointing; it's even okay if a test result isn't what you'd hoped for. I think of this as the state of *wishlessness*, a word I first learned from Ayya Khema. It's a tall order to let go completely, but simply imagining it inspires me to let go a little. Then it's easier to let go a little more, and then a lot. And every once in a while, I let go completely and, momentarily, bask in the glow of that blessed state of freedom and serenity that is equanimity.

Giving in instead of giving up. The challenge with equanimity practice is to not let accepting things the way they are slip into indifference, because indifference is a subtle aversion to life as it is. Indifference turns the serene *giving in* of "Things are as they are" into the mental pain of *giving up*, as in "Things are as they are—so who cares?"

Giving up can make us feel like failures. We may begin to see ourselves as mentally weak and undisciplined. This is disheartening and tends to give rise to the misery of self-blame—that inner critic again. By contrast, giving in is a type of surrender. I think of it as sweet surrender. It's the act of accepting what we cannot change and then looking for how to live a fulfilling life within our limitations.

Here are some examples of how you might turn giving up into giving in:

Giving up: "I don't care what happens; chronic illness has ruined my life."

Giving in: "Yes, I'm frustrated and sad at times that I'm not in good health, but a good life can take many forms, so let me think about what I can do that's within my limitations."

Giving up: "Because I couldn't visit with my friend for very long today, it wasn't worth seeing her at all."

Giving in: "Dwelling on what I couldn't do makes me feel sad and even angry. The fact is, I had a good time while it lasted. Now I have to rest."

Giving up: "I hate being sick. I hate being in pain. I hate being depressed. I give up."

Giving in: "Treating chronic illness as the enemy drains what little energy I have. Everyone's life has its challenges; this one is mine. I give in to it and will try to find a measure of peace within these less than ideal circumstances."

A medication I was prescribed in 2016 caused me to become clinically depressed. For several months, I had a front row seat for the mental suffering that accompanies giving up. I didn't want to do anything. I lost interest in the activities I used to enjoy—writing, crocheting, tending to my bonsai trees. I couldn't be bothered. I also had a recurring feeling of dread about the present and the future. It was a new experience for me, and it was not a pleasant one. (I've joked with Tony that it's a good thing my publisher proposed this new edition of *How to Be Sick* after I'd stopped taking that medication and the depression had lifted because, otherwise, I would have said no.) Because of my experience with this medication, I'm now keenly aware of how hard it is for people with chronic depression to change that "giving up" feeling into the peace and contentment of "giving in." I hope this section has made it possible.

Accepting loss. Facing losses that feel overwhelming—from lost health to lost friends to lost livelihood—deeply challenges our cultivation of equanimity. But we can sometimes find teachings and practices in the most unexpected of places. One day I was watching an interview on TV with the actress Susan Saint James. Three weeks before the interview, her fourteen-year-old son, Teddy, was killed in a plane crash. Her husband and another son were seriously injured and several of the crew members died. In the interview, Saint James talked about how close she was to Teddy because he was her youngest child and the only one still living at home; due to his work as the head of NBC Sports, her husband, Dick Ebersol, was gone much of the time. She said that she and Teddy were like roommates and had become best friends.

Then, emanating deep calm and acceptance, she made this most astonishing comment: "His was a life that lasted fourteen years." I gasped. Could I make that statement with such equanimity should one of my children or grandchildren die? I still don't know the answer to that question. But Susan Saint James's words and the serenity with which she spoke them entered my heart that day. Ever since, when I find myself in grief and despair over the many losses I've had to face due to chronic illness, her words are my equanimity practice.

When I feel myself mourning my lost career as a law professor or a lost friendship, I say to myself, "This was a career that lasted twenty years" or "This was a friendship that lasted twenty-five years." If I feel overwhelmed by the loss of my health and its consequences, I say to myself, "This was a body that was illness-free long enough to be active in raising my children and to not be a burden to them when they were young; to be a part of their weddings; to teach and be of personal support to many law students; to travel and keep company with Tony out in the world."

Inspired by Susan Saint James's courage, which reinforces the teachings of the Buddha that I've learned, I'm able to say these equanimity phrases without bitterness. I can even be genuinely grateful for those years. When overcome with the losses you've encountered, whether you are chronically ill or the caregiver for a loved one who is chronically ill, I encourage you to try the equanimity practice I cobbled together from the words of a remarkable woman facing the most devastating loss I can imagine.

This section of the book has covered the four sublime states: kindness, compassion, empathetic joy, and equanimity. The goal is to cultivate them until they become the natural response to whatever you encounter in life. As you undertake these practices, I recommend that you keep what the Korean Zen Master Ko Bong called a "Try Mind." I love this idea because implicit in Try Mind is "Forgiving Mind": "I tried to wish that person well today and I tried to feel equanimous about my circumstances, but I just couldn't do it. That's okay. I'll try again tomorrow."

Cultivating the sublime states opens the door to the peace and well-being we all seek. May you come to greet all of life's experiences with an open heart.

Turnarounds and Transformations

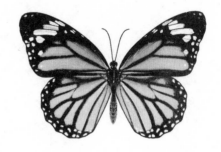

10

Getting Off the Wheel of Suffering

Nothing whatsoever should be clung to.
—BUDDHADASA BHIKKHU

MANY TEACHERS SUGGEST starting Buddhist practice by learning how to meditate, but I was an academic and so, as was my habit, I hit the books first and did some research on the subject. So great was my need to put scholarship first that soon after becoming interested in Buddhism in 1992 I researched and wrote a twenty-page paper, complete with footnotes that referenced over three dozen books. I titled it "Introduction to Buddhism." Given that I can't recall giving this little piece of scholarship to anyone, I appear to have been introducing myself to Buddhism.

I started my study with a book we already owned: *What the Buddha Taught*, written in 1959 by the Sri Lankan monk and scholar Walpola Rahula. In 1992, when I took it off the bookshelf, this work was still considered by many to be the seminal guide for introducing Westerners to Buddhism. It was not an easy read, especially in contrast to the large number of user-friendly books on Buddhism available today. Rahula's use of phrases such as

99

"dependent origination," "conditioned genesis," and "cessation of volitional formations" had my mind spinning. When I reached Rahula's discussion of the wheel of suffering, I might well have been derailed in this new spiritual pursuit had I not employed a strategy that had served me well in my studies: I skipped it and moved to a teaching that was more accessible.

Years later, my Buddhist practice well established, I tackled that teaching again through the writings of Ayya Khema and S. N. Goenka, and it began to make sense. *When the Iron Eagle Flies,* by Ayya Khema, and *The Art of Living: Vipassana Meditation as Taught by S. N. Goenka,* by William Hart, were particularly helpful.

The Buddha's teaching on the wheel of suffering describes a series of twelve conditions that give rise to suffering. With the caveat that this will not be a comprehensive nor scholarly analysis, I'm going to jump into the middle of the series and explain how I use these teachings as a practical tool to help alleviate the mental suffering that accompanies chronic illness.

As we go through life, we repeatedly encounter mental and physical contacts through our six senses. (Buddhism treats the mind as a sixth sense, along with sight, smell, touch, taste, and hearing.) We experience these contacts as pleasant, unpleasant, or (less frequently) neutral sensations. If the experience of the contact is *pleasant*, we want more of it. If the experience of the contact is *unpleasant*, we want it to go away, which is simply another form of desire—the desire for it to go away—usually referred to in Buddhism as aversion. In chapter 3, when I described the second noble truth as "Want/Don't-Want Mind," I was referring to our desire for pleasant experiences and our aversion to unpleasant ones. (To be honest, "want" and "don't-want" sum up the two mental states I find myself in a good part of the day!)

Having reacted with desire or aversion to what we've come in contact with through our six senses, the mind sticks like glue to the desire or the aversion. This "place" on the wheel of suffering is varyingly referred to as *clinging* or *attachment* and is Want/Don't-Want Mind's close cousin. Once clinging or attachment takes hold, the sense of a solid self arises—as if the glue has dried. In short, we are reborn moment to moment into self-identities we create by clinging or attaching to the objects of our desires and aversions.

We then have to live out the consequences of the birth (or rebirth, if you like) that we've taken in the moment. Here's a simple example. Someone merges in front of us in traffic even though we have the right-of-way. Note that this contact with the world involves more than one sense: the eyes see the car merge, the ears hear the car move, the sixth sense thinks, "He's cutting in front of me even though I have the right-of-way." The part of the contact involving the mind is experienced as unpleasant. Before we can stop ourselves, we react with aversion to the unpleasantness. In fact, we can't shake the aversion. It takes hold of us, sticking like glue, putting us right on course for "becoming" and being "reborn" that very moment as a cranky person. And there you have it: dukkha—from the Four Noble Truths.

The good news is that we can break this cycle before we reach that place of suffering by becoming mindful right at the moment before an unpleasant sensation gives rise to the desire that things be other than they are. S. N. Goenka refers to this as "learning to observe [sensations] objectively." He says that between the contact and the reaction to a pleasant or unpleasant sensation—a reaction in the form of desire or aversion—stands a crucial step: "When we learn to observe sensation without reacting in craving [desire] and aversion, the cause of suffering does not arise and suffering ceases."

That split second between the experience of a pleasant or

unpleasant sensation and the arising of desire for more of the former or aversion to the latter is the doorway out—our opportunity to get off the wheel of suffering. We can't avoid the arising of a sensation after a contact—touching a hot stove is going to feel unpleasant. But Ayya Khema says that the practice is to see that sensation as just a sensation without owning it. After all, she says, if we really "owned" our sensations in the sense of being fully able to control them, we'd never let those sensations be anything but pleasant! This is also what S. N. Goenka means when he says we should learn to observe sensations objectively.

When someone merges in front of us in traffic even though we have the right-of-way, we can simply observe that the mental sensations of judgment and aversion feel unpleasant and leave the experience at that—without reacting to it as anything more than one of the thousands of momentary contacts we encounter every day. If we do this, not only will we become attuned to the truth of impermanence, but also, suffering will not arise, and before we know it, we've moved on to the next contact of the day, which might be a sympathetic smile from another driver.

This takes us to a practice I developed that combines the teachings of the wheel of suffering with the four sublime states—even though they may appear to be an unlikely partnership.

Practicing with the Wheel of Suffering and the Four Sublime States

The idea for this practice began with a teaching from the wise and wonderful Sylvia Boorstein, whom I mentioned earlier. Sylvia is one of Spirit Rock's founding teachers. In her book *Happiness Is an Inside Job,* she tells the story of how she and her husband, Seymour, were visiting a ski resort in Europe. As Sylvia watched people learning to ski, she recalled all the times she and Seymour had tackled the slopes together before reaching the age where it was no longer safe for them to do so. When her mind began to "wobble," as she puts it (my wobble would have been straight to the unpleasant mental feeling of envy), she looked around at all the fun people were having and suddenly felt great delight in their joy, especially that of a little girl who was just learning to ski. And so with her wisdom mind, Sylvia turned that approaching negative mental state into the sublime state of empathetic joy.

Shortly after I read this chapter in Sylvia's book, Tony and I were talking about how we seem to be hard-wired to experience contact as pleasant, unpleasant, or neutral. This includes both physical and mental contact: I can no more turn touching a hot stove into a pleasant experience than I can turn hearing a racist comment into one. The question for me becomes whether I can get off the wheel of suffering at that point, before the unpleasant experience of something such as a racist comment turns into aversion—the "don't-want" side of desire. Once I react with aversion, clinging isn't far behind, and before I know it I've completed going around the wheel of suffering and have been "reborn" as a person so full of anger that I'm unable to take wise action to counter the comment.

I had been mulling over both Sylvia's skiing chapter and this discussion with Tony when the time came for me to try to nap. I lay in bed, my body aching with flu-like symptoms, my heart pounding with wired fatigue. Of course, I was experiencing this as an unpleasant physical sensation. My mind began its usual movement—Sylvia's "wobble"—from the experience of the unpleasantness to aversion, when I realized how to find that doorway out that S. N. Goenka and others talk about. In other words, I found a way to break the vicious cycle of suffering. I did it by consciously moving my mind toward one of the four sublime states.

As I lay in bed, the flu-like symptoms were indeed physically unpleasant. But instead of mindlessly allowing aversion to arise as I had done thousands of times in the past, I realized I had a choice of where to put my mind. So I consciously moved my mind to metta by being kind to myself, silently repeating, "Dear sweet, innocent body, may you feel better soon." Directing this kindness toward my own body was my doorway out of the wheel of suffering. I was free from aversion to my illness and from all that can follow from that aversion—for example, becoming and being reborn as a bitter and resentful person.

Of course, I was so conditioned to moving straight to aversion or desire that this breakthrough didn't mean I no longer had to work at all this. Every day I have to work on learning to observe sensations objectively, and sometimes I don't make it out that door. But I practice hard at it.

I practice by first becoming mindful that, yes, this bodily sickness feels unpleasant. Then I consciously move my mind to whatever sublime state works for me at that moment. So I may move to metta practice—kindness—as in chapter 7. Or I may evoke compassion for myself, silently saying, "It's so hard to feel this sick. It's hard to feel under attack by some mystery virus and not be able to find a treatment that works." Often as I say this, I pet one arm with the hand of the other. Sometimes my mind inclines toward equanimity and I silently say, "This is how it is. My body is sick. It's okay. This is just how my life is." Recently I've developed the ability to cultivate empathetic joy so that, as I lie in bed experiencing unpleasant bodily sensations, I'm able to feel happy, even if just a little, for those who are in good health.

I also use empathetic joy in the same way Sylvia did. When I'm not able to visit with my family in the front of the house and I experience it as unpleasant, instead of getting stuck in aversion and all the suffering that inevitably follows, I intentionally try to feel joyful that they're able to spend this time with one another.

I have used this practice of combining awareness of the wheel of suffering with the four sublime states to help me through the most difficult of circumstances. For example, I had a period of two days and nights when I stopped sleeping. It wasn't insomnia. The malaise and the oppressive, heart-pounding fatigue of my illness were too strong to allow my body to fall asleep in the same way as someone in pain can't sleep. When people who are well have a couple of sleepless nights, they don't feel good during the day, but they can function. For me, a good night's sleep is only partially restorative, so you can imagine how not sleeping at all affected me.

During those two sleepless nights, my previous reaction would have been to go straight from the unpleasant physical sensation to aversion followed by misery. I would have lain in bed getting increasingly frustrated and angry at my body. Instead, I consciously moved my mind among the four sublime states.

At one A.M., I treated myself with kindness: "Rest as best you can, sweet body."

At two A.M., I felt empathetic joy: "I'm glad that others are able to sleep tonight."

At three A.M., I evoked compassion for myself: "It's so hard to lie in bed, needing to sleep but not being able to."

At four A.M., I cultivated equanimity: "This is how things are; my body is not able to sleep right now."

On the third night, I slept.

I'm convinced that using these practices to keep the unpleasant sensations from turning into frustration and aversion kept

Getting Off the Wheel of Suffering 105

my symptoms from increasing more than they already had and eventually allowed the flare-up to subside. I'm so grateful that these two Buddhist practices teamed up to help me through that difficult time.

11

Tonglen: Spinning Straw into Gold

O that my monk's robe
were wide enough
to gather up all
the suffering people
in this floating world.
—RYOKAN

TONGLEN IS a compassion practice that comes from the Tibetan Buddhist tradition. Nonetheless, the above Zen poem by Ryokan captures for me the essence of tonglen. Of course, they are both inspired by the example of the Buddha.

When I first got sick, it didn't take long for me to accumulate a collection of healing CDs from a variety of spiritual traditions. They had one thing in common: I was instructed to breathe *in* peaceful and healing thoughts and images, and to breathe *out* my mental and physical suffering. In tonglen practice, however, the instruction is to do the opposite. We breathe *in* the suffering of the world and then, as we breathe *out*, we release that suffering and offer others whatever measure of kindness, compassion, and peace of mind we have to give. It's a counterintuitive practice, which is why the Buddhist nun and teacher Pema Chödrön says that tonglen reverses ego's logic.

Tonglen practice was brought to Tibet from India in the eleventh century as part of a group of teachings known as the "seven points of mind training," a collection of fifty-nine "slogans" for practicing the path of compassion. The practice of tonglen is described in this slogan: train in taking and sending alternately; put them on the breath.

Those two phrases don't give us a lot of guidance, but for hundreds of years this slogan, along with the other fifty-eight, has been a favorite subject for commentary by Tibetan masters who flesh out the meaning of each slogan. Tonglen, literally translated as "giving and receiving," has become "Breathe in the suffering of others; breathe out thoughts of kindness, compassion, and peace." We are, in effect, breathing out the sublime states of mind introduced in earlier chapters.

I had learned tonglen practice before getting sick, but I didn't use it very often. Now it's one of my principal compassion practices. My bond with tonglen occurred on the first day I returned to work, six months after getting sick in Paris.

Like everyone else around me, I couldn't believe I wasn't well enough to continue with my profession, at least on a part-time basis. So a half-hour before my scheduled class, Tony dropped me off at the front door of the law school. It was the second week of January 2002. I took the elevator up one floor to my office. I was to teach Marital Property to second- and third-year students. As soon as I sat down in my office chair, I knew I was too sick to be there. I began to panic, so I lay down on a couch in the office. Unexpectedly, my thoughts turned to the millions of people who must go to work every day even though they're chronically ill. I realized that many of these people were in a worse position than

I was—if they didn't go to work, they wouldn't be able to pay the rent or buy food for their families.

I'd been in the workforce for dozens of years but had never before thought about people being forced to work while not feeling well. As I was contemplating this, I began to breathe in their suffering, which, as a chronically ill person myself, now included my own suffering. Then I breathed out what kindness, compassion, and peace of mind I had to give. To my surprise, the panic subsided and was replaced with a feeling of deep connection to all these people. Even more astonishing was the realization that, as sick and in pain as I was at that moment and as preoccupied as I was about the task awaiting me in less than ten minutes, I was still able to send some thoughts of kindness, compassion, and peace to others on the out-breath.

A few minutes later, I arose from the couch, took a chair with me, and, for the first time in twenty years, taught a class while sitting down. For the next two and a half years of part-time teaching, I used tonglen in my office, followed by adrenaline in the classroom, to get me through the workweek. Only Tony saw the devastating effect that continuing to work had on me as I went straight from the car to the bed and stayed there until the next class I had to teach. When I think of those years, tonglen and that couch in my office are inseparable in my mind. I don't know how I would have survived without both.

Inspired by what had happened that first day back at work, I began to use tonglen all the time. I'd use it while waiting for the results of medical tests related to my ongoing illness. It took me out of my small world—out of exclusive focus on my illness—and connected me with all the people caught up in the medical system who were anxiously waiting to hear the results of tests. It never failed to amaze me that no matter how worried I was, there were always some good wishes, some compassion, and some serenity inside me to send out to others in the same situation. Finding our own storehouse of kindness and compassion is the wonder of tonglen practice. Gradually, the fear over my test results diminished and I was able to wait with equanimity to see what the world had in store for me next. And, of course, some years later, I relied on tonglen to help me cope with the anxiety of waiting for test results related to the breast cancer.

I love that tonglen is a two-for-one compassion practice. The formal instruction is to breathe in the suffering of others and breathe out thoughts of kindness, compassion, and peace. But the effect of repeated practice is that we connect with our own suffering, anguish, stress, and discomfort. So as we breathe in the suffering of someone who is in the midst of a similar struggle, we are also breathing in our own suffering over that struggle as well. As we breathe out whatever measure of kindness, compassion, and peace of mind we have to give, we are offering those sublime states to ourselves, too. *All* beings are included.

A day did come when I reached my limit with tonglen. I tried the practice on Thanksgiving Day, two and a half years after I got sick, while lying in my bedroom and listening to the sound of my family chatting and laughing in the front of the house. I tried breathing in the sadness and sorrow of all the people who were in the same house as their family on Thanksgiving but weren't well enough to join the festivities. It was too much; I couldn't hold everyone's suffering without crying. So I cried.

But four years later, in similar circumstances, the practice was tremendously helpful to me. It was a measure of how tonglen had slowly worked its magic. My second grandchild, Camden Bodhi, was born in September 2007, and I planned a welcoming party

110 *Turnarounds and Transformations*

for her that, as it turned out, I could not attend. When I set the plan in motion in the spring, I was halfway through a yearlong experimental antiviral treatment that appeared to be working. But six months later, on the day of the party, I was too sick to take the hour-long trip to Berkeley. I lay in bed that day thinking about friends and family who had gathered to celebrate my granddaughter's birth, and I was overcome with sorrow.

First I tried empathetic joy—feeling good about all the fun everyone was having at the celebration. It helped, but I continued to feel sad and disheartened by my inability to attend, by thoughts about the good time I was missing, and by the feeling that I had let others down. So I turned to tonglen. I breathed in the suffering of all those who were unable to be with their families on special days of celebration. As I did this, I was aware I was breathing in my own sadness and sorrow, but unlike that Thanksgiving Day, I was able to hold the suffering—to care for it—without feeling overcome by it. I then breathed out thoughts of kindness, compassion, and peace for them and for myself. The connection I felt with all those people was powerful and moving.

If you feel hesitant to try tonglen for fear that breathing in other people's suffering could overwhelm you, you're not alone. Here's the response given by the eco-philosopher and Buddhist scholar Joanna Macy when that very concern was raised at a Spirit Rock workshop. First she reassured the woman asking the question that her capacity to hold others' suffering was greater than she imagined. Then she said, "If you really could alleviate all the suffering in the world by breathing it in, wouldn't you?"

Of course, this is a hypothetical ideal and so is not a realistic assessment of the effect of practicing tonglen. Indeed, at times we may cry in response to breathing in the suffering in the world, but these are tears of compassion—a perfectly appropriate response. And those moments when we *can* hold the suffering of the world on the in-breath and breathe out whatever kindness, compassion, and peace of mind we have to give are like turning straw into gold.

12

With Our Thoughts We Make the World
AN APPRECIATION OF BYRON KATIE

*In our everyday life, our thinking is 99 percent
self-centered. "Why do I have suffering?
Why do I have trouble?"*
—SHUNRYU SUZUKI

SEVERAL YEARS BEFORE I became chronically ill, I attended a retreat in Northern California led by Ayya Khema. In it, she gave a talk on the nature of thought. According to my notes, she said at one point: "Thoughts are just there, like the air around us. They arise but are arbitrary and not reliable. Most of them are just rubbish, but we believe them anyway."

I took her words to heart and, before getting sick, had become quite adept at applying this teaching. Especially while in formal meditation, I could watch a thought arise in the mind, treat it as impersonal energy, and let it pass through. I knew I couldn't control the content of thoughts that arose, but I also knew it wasn't the content that led to suffering. Suffering arose when I "believed" the thought—when I believed it was a valid reflection of reality. I knew, for example, that the thought "My Torts class won't go well today" didn't mean that the class wouldn't be just fine. Believing a thought is another way of saying that we're clinging to it, continuing to go round and round on the wheel of suffering.

By the time the Parisian Flu hit, I had a good understanding of the nature of thoughts and the circumstances under which they gave rise to suffering. But put me in the sickbed all day and suddenly my thoughts seemed anything but impersonal. As for Ayya Khema's statement that thoughts are arbitrary and not reliable, I now believed every one of them held the force of Absolute Truth:

"I'll never feel joy again."
"No doctor wants to treat me."
"All my friends have abandoned me."
"I've ruined Tony's life."

Thoughts and suffering were now marching hand in hand in my life.

Feeling overwhelmed by this barrage of stressful thoughts, I turned to the Buddha for help. His words as recorded in a small book called the *Dhammapada* came to mind: "With our thoughts we make the world."

With my thoughts I had made a world of suffering to live in. And the thoughts had a stranglehold on me because I believed they were true—that I *was* ruining Tony's life, that I *wouldn't* feel joy again. In confronting the suffering that my thoughts were causing, I was helped by an inspiring teacher named Byron Katie. Katie, as everyone calls her, encourages us to question the validity of our stressful thoughts. I highly recommend her books and her website. Using what she calls "The Work," or "inquiry," she sets forth a five-step method for revealing the suffering that follows when we believe our thoughts. Along with the Buddha's teachings, Byron Katie's inquiry has been the most powerful tool I've found to help with the challenges of being chronically ill.

Inquiry Practice

When I became housebound, it wasn't long before I started to worry about the fate of my friendships. Yet instead of examining the possible reasons why friends might not be visiting, I kept thinking over and over, "My friends should not stop coming to see me." Each time the thought arose, it was accompanied by hurt and anger. This particular thought became an ever-present source of stress and suffering in my life until I began to use Byron Katie's five-step inquiry practice to question the validity of the thought. Here's how it works.

In the first step, we ask whether the thought is true; in this case I answered, "Yes, it is true that my friends should not stop coming to see me."

In the second step, we ask whether we're absolutely sure that it's true. On this, I was not as certain: "*Am* I *absolutely* sure it's true? Hmm. Maybe this requires a bit more investigation . . ."

The third step in questioning the validity of a stressful thought is to notice how we feel when we believe the thought. When I believed the thought "My friends should not stop coming to see me," I felt angry and hurt, almost as if I were being wounded physically.

The fourth step is to reflect on who we'd be without the thought. I closed my eyes and imagined who I'd be . . . and my answer was, "I'd be living this day as it unfolds—seeing what it brings, instead of being focused on who may or may not visit." Without the stressful thought "My friends should not stop coming to see me," I felt liberated, as if a heavy burden had been lifted—the burden of constantly worrying about the state of my friendships.

Then comes the counterintuitive fifth step, when Katie asks us to come up with a "turnaround." The turnaround is a statement of the stressful thought in a way that's opposite from its original expression. There's no one "right" turnaround; we are to find one that we can work with. Once we settle on a turnaround, we're to come up with at least three reasons why it might be true.

For the turnaround, I tried saying, "My friends *should* stop coming to see me." At first that sounded absurd, but the more I considered this turnaround, the more I was able to see that there were genuine reasons why my friends might not be visiting. Many people are uncomfortable around others who are unwell—they might be afraid they'll develop health problems, or perhaps seeing someone who is sick or in pain reminds them of their own mortality. It's also possible that they're currently facing medical problems of their own, making it impossible for them to be in touch with me right now. Or they might not be visiting because they think it will be too hard on me, or maybe they don't know what to talk to me about because they're worried I'll feel bad if they share the fun and rewarding things they're doing while I'm stuck at home. In addition, people get caught up in the busyness of their lives; they often barely have time to spend with their own families.

Working on the turnaround in this way led to two other unexpected insights. First, while generating all these possible reasons why friends might not be visiting, it dawned on me for the first time that just because they weren't visiting—or even calling me—didn't mean they weren't thinking kind thoughts about me and hoping that I'd get better. Over the years, hadn't there been people I knew who were struggling with a health problem, people I could have contacted but didn't? Absolutely.

Second, I realized that the reasons friends weren't coming to see me had to do with what was going on in their minds, not mine. I can't control the thoughts that arise in my *own* mind. What made me think I could control what my friends were thinking? No wonder when, in the fourth step, I reflected on who I'd be without

116   *Turnarounds and Transformations*

the stressful thought, I felt as if a heavy burden had been lifted. As the Buddha said, with our thoughts we make our world. I had created a bitter and resentful world.

Working with Byron Katie's inquiry showed me that I had spun so many emotionally fraught tales about why friends weren't visiting that I hadn't stopped to examine what the true reasons might be. It wasn't my friends who were the source of my suffering; it was my own unexamined thinking about them. That wound I was feeling turned out to be self-inflicted. Now it could begin to heal. I stopped blaming friends for not visiting and I no longer assumed they didn't care about me.

I use Byron Katie's inquiry all the time. I even used it when I was stuck-like-glue on a stressful thought about her! Tony was planning to attend a daylong session with her at Spirit Rock. I really wanted to go. I felt as if I knew her personally from her books and from videos. On her website, I had watched her use one-on-one dialogues to guide people through the "four questions and a turnaround."

So, as Katie would have suggested, I wrote down the thought that was causing me so much stress: "I really want to go to Spirit Rock on Saturday to see Katie." Then I subjected the thought to her five-step process. Not only was it true that I wanted to go but, unlike my example with friends not visiting, this time I was sure it was "absolutely true." Katie says that starting with these two questions—Is the thought true? Are we absolutely sure it's true?—forces us to commit one way or the other. Then we can watch how the mind acts to defend our response: "Don't tell me I might not want to go to Spirit Rock. I absolutely do!"

Then I moved to the third question and asked how I felt when I believed the thought "I really want to go to Spirit Rock on Saturday to see Katie." I felt anger and resentment. I felt like a victim in an unfair world. But when I moved to the fourth question and asked who I'd be without the thought, I immediately saw that I'd be a person living in the present moment, which happened to be a beautifully sunbathed Tuesday—days away from the Saturday event.

Working through these four questions was helpful, but, as can happen, the stressful thought persisted until I got to the magical turnaround. I turned the thought around to "I don't want to see Katie on Saturday." Then, following Katie's instructions, I looked for at least three reasons why the turnaround might be true. I came up with five. First, it would take me a week, maybe several, to recover from the trip. Second, the event was going to be extremely crowded, so I might not be able to find a comfortable place to sit or lie down. Third, I might catch a cold or the flu from someone who was there. Fourth, by seeing Katie in person I might not improve my inquiry skills any more than I would by continuing to watch her videos on my computer. Fifth, she could be a big disappointment! (I know from watching her video dialogues with others that Katie would have enjoyed that last turnaround.)

After putting all this down on paper—as she suggests we do because of the power of the written word—I was fully content not to go on Saturday. I had let go of the stressful thought and it never returned, even when I saw Tony off to the event.

One day I wrote down a thought that, understandably, was a great source of suffering: "I hate being sick."

It was true, and I was sure it was *absolutely* true. How did I feel when I believed the thought? Bitter, frustrated, singled out by the world. Who would I be without the thought? I'd be a woman, lying on a comfortable bed in a quiet room, enjoying the exquisite play of sunlight on the tail of the squirrel who was visible outside my window. Katie says she isn't telling us to give up the stressful thought but to drop it for long enough to see who we'd be without it.

Then I turned the thought around: "I love being sick."

Could I possibly come up with three reasons why this turnaround might be true? I thought not, but I let ink from my pen flow onto the page anyway. When I was finished, I'd come up with twelve reasons. Here's what I wrote, unedited, and in the order I wrote it:

1. I don't answer to an alarm clock.
2. I have the perfect excuse to avoid events and people I don't want to be with.
3. I have lots of time to be with Tony and Rusty, our dog.
4. I'm getting to know Bridgett, my daughter-in-law, really well for the first time.
5. My life is pretty quiet and peaceful.
6. I'm never stuck in traffic.
7. I don't have to work.
8. There's nothing I have to read or study.
9. My to-do list is very short.
10. Most of my day is unplanned, so in summer, I can lie down in the backyard before it gets too hot and in winter, wait until it warms up to do so.
11. I've met some people I wouldn't have otherwise known.
12. Being home sick allowed our elderly dog, Winnie, to live another year since, in that last year, she couldn't be home alone.

I can't say that since performing this inquiry I haven't again believed the thought "I hate being sick" and suffered as a consequence. I have dozens of times—this work is not necessarily about ridding oneself of stressful thoughts but rather about examining their validity. But the work I did that day on "I hate being sick" is right there, on paper, and rereading it is always helpful.

Then came the day when I tackled this stressful thought: "I am sick."

I was surprised at the number of genuine reasons why the turnaround was true: "I am not sick."

My mind isn't sick—I'm able to do this inquiry. My heart isn't sick—I can express love and be of help to others. Not all my body is sick—I can walk, I can type, I can see the birds, I can hear music. I came away from that exercise truly not feeling like a sick person. In fact, I realized that the more I believed the thought, "I am sick," the sicker I felt.

By offering us a systematic method for examining thoughts that are a source of dukkha (suffering, stress, dissatisfaction with our lives), Byron Katie's inquiry takes us to the Buddha's first and second noble truths: we create dukkha when we believe we *must* get our way. I wanted friends to visit. I wanted to go to Spirit Rock to see Katie. I didn't want to be sick. Subjecting stressful thoughts like these to Katie's "four questions and a turnaround" gives us a tool for making peace with our life as it is.

13

The Present Moment as a Refuge

When we settle into the present moment,
we can see beauties and wonders right before our eyes—
a newborn baby, the sun rising in the sky.

—THICH NHAT HANH

WHEN PEOPLE FIRST realize they have a chronic condition that's going to severely restrict their activities, they'll try just about anything to get their old lives back: off-label use of prescription drugs, homeopathic medicine, esoteric mind-therapy techniques, nutritional supplements, oxygen chambers. When the Parisian Flu settled into a chronic illness, I scoured the Internet looking for possible treatments. (I have a large box that I refer to as the "Box of Rejected Supplements.")

My online wanderings revealed that many people, regardless of their religious affiliation, find that starting a meditation practice is the most helpful treatment they've tried. So, Buddhist or not, many people turn *to* meditation when they become chronically ill. This devoted Buddhist, however, turned away from it.

When I got sick, I had a mindfulness meditation practice that I'd been doing consistently for ten years. I meditated twice a day for forty-five minutes each time, following the traditional instruction to rest my attention on the physical sensation of the breath as it comes in and goes out of my body—sometimes called "following the breath." When my mind wandered to other things—perhaps to thoughts about all I had to accomplish the next day—I'd gently bring it back to following the breath again. The purpose of mindfulness meditation is to keep returning to the experience of the present moment. (More detailed instructions can be found online, in Buddhist books, at meditation centers, and at many medical clinics in the form of mindfulness-based stress and pain reduction programs.)

I was so disciplined and stubborn about my meditation practice that it had become part of our family lore to recall—and to tease me about—how on our daughter's wedding day, I still managed to get in my two formal sittings. What made this remarkable was that, although Mara and Brad lived in Washington, DC, the wedding was in Davis, where Mara grew up. She and Brad arrived in Davis two days before the festivities. I have never been one to throw parties; Tony and I had twelve people at our wedding. Nevertheless, here I was, putting on a traditional wedding for over 150 people! Needless to say, I was overwhelmed by my responsibilities on the wedding day. But the family knew: whatever else happens on this day, Mom is going to meditate, not once, but twice.

At the Spirit Rock retreat in July 2001, when I awoke on the third day and realized that some form of the Parisian Flu had returned, I raised it at my next teacher interview. I reported that I found it difficult to meditate because I was physically ill. I was told that being sick was the very best time to meditate because it would prepare me for when I was approaching death. I should "follow my breath" and note the illness-related body sensations as they arose. I returned to my room and lay on the bed, trying over and over to meditate, but the sickly body sensations were too unpleasant for me to keep my attention on. I couldn't do it on the retreat and, upon returning home, to the surprise of my family, I discarded that ten-year meditation practice that we all thought was set in stone. I felt like a failure whenever I'd read online how helpful meditation was to people who were chronically ill. But when I would try, the discomfort of my illness was overwhelming.

It took me fourteen years to take up mindfulness meditation again, but I do it differently now. I no longer have hard and fast rules. I lie on the bed and pay attention to the physical sensation of the breath as it comes in and goes out of my body—one of many meditation techniques. This anchors me in the present moment. Of course, my attention drifts now and then, usually to thoughts about the past or the future. When I become aware this has happened, I gently return my attention to the sensation of the in- and out-breath. I do this for between twenty and forty-five minutes. And if I'm too sick or in too much pain to meditate on any given day, I don't do it. Allowing myself this flexibility works for me.

In the years since I've been chronically ill, more essential to me than formal meditation has been *mindfulness outside of meditation*. *Mindfulness* refers to paying attention to your present-moment experience. It's as simple as that. There's no belief system associated with mindfulness, even as it was originally taught by the Buddha. For me, fully engaging my present-moment experience has become a refuge from the exhaustion created by constant discursive thinking, whether I'm ruminating about the past, worrying about the future, or judging what's going on around and inside me.

I'm aware that the word *mindfulness* has become so pervasive in our culture that it can feel as if it's lost its freshness and even its meaning. My goal in this chapter is to make it come alive again by offering specific ideas, rather than just telling you, "Be mindful

The Present Moment as a Refuge 123

of everything you do." And so here are five simple practices that are easy to try. See which ones resonate with you.

Describe Your Present-Moment Experience Objectively

From my daughter, Mara, I learned a remarkable practice. It comes from Byron Katie. Mara was listening to a podcast of Oprah Winfrey interviewing Katie on the radio show *Oprah and Friends*. Katie was sharing a story about her daughter, who, years ago, had problems with alcohol and drugs. Her daughter would go out at night in her car and, in the early hours of the morning, Katie would sit and wait for her daughter to return. The later it got, the more stressful Katie's thoughts became. She would imagine her daughter had been raped, or that she'd been in an auto accident and was dead or was lying injured on the road in agony with no one to help her. Then one early morning, as the same thoughts began to arise again, Katie realized that the only thing that was true for sure was this: "Woman in chair, waiting for her beloved daughter."

Mara heard this story and knew it contained a gem, because she started to free her own mind of stressful thoughts and ground herself in the moment by using whatever version of Katie's words applied. In fact, Mara happened to share this story with me because the day before had been a particularly stressful one for her, physically and emotionally (an emergency trip to the dentist for my granddaughter Malia was but one of the highlights). Mara said that as she was lying in bed that night, trying to read, stressful thoughts about the day kept spinning around in her mind. It was as if she were reliving the day over and over. (We've all done this, haven't we?) Then she said to herself, "Woman lying in bed, reading a book." Suddenly she was, well, just a woman lying in bed, reading a book! She'd brought herself out of painful ruminating about the past and into the present moment.

I've found that this practice works best in the context of chronic illness if you're careful to do what Mara did—make your description objective; that is, leave out emotionally charged words, such as *horrible* or *unbearable*. For example, instead of saying, "Sitting in my car with horrible neck pain" or "On my bed, feeling unbearably depressed," simply say, "Sitting in my car with neck pain" or "On my bed, feeling depressed." Leaving out the emotional descriptors minimizes the likelihood that you'll start spinning stressful stories that will only make you feel worse, stories such as how the neck pain or the depression *will never go away.* As we know from chapter 4, everything changes. No physical or mental symptom is set in stone.

I used Byron Katie's practice for the first time the very day after Mara shared it with me. I was caught up in a repeating round of stressful thoughts about the previous day. I was blaming myself for not having been more disciplined about the amount of time I'd spent socializing with a friend who had come over. Of course, it's not a bad idea to examine the effects of oversocializing on our symptoms, but blaming ourselves and feeling guilty about something that's already happened is not constructive.

"It's your own fault that you feel so sick today," I thought for the dozenth time, at which point I looked up and saw my face in the mirror of the bathroom sink and said, "Woman on stool, brushing her teeth." It was a magical moment. It broke the hold these stressful thoughts had on me. Just to be sure, I repeated (to use Katie's words) the only thing that was true for sure, "Woman on stool, brushing her teeth." And I smiled, because being in the present moment is a relief indeed!

Try Thich Nhat Hanh's Mindfulness Exercises

In *The Miracle of Mindfulness,* the Vietnamese Zen master Thich Nhat Hanh offers several exercises for staying mindful of the present moment as we engage in activities of everyday life, from brushing our teeth to making the bed to washing the dishes. Many of them start with the instruction to "half-smile"—a wonderful practice in itself. Try a half-smile and see how your mind and body immediately relax and how a touch of serenity arises. Here are two of Thich Nhat Hanh's mindfulness exercises, which you can easily apply in your own life:

> *Half-smile while listening to music.* Listen to a piece of music for two or three minutes. Pay attention to the words, melody, rhythm, and sentiments. Smile while watching your inhalations and exhalations.

> *Mindfulness while making tea.* Prepare a pot of tea. Do each movement slowly, in mindfulness. Do not let one detail of your movements go by without being mindful of it. Know that your hand lifts the pot by its handle, know that you are pouring the fragrant warm tea into the cup. Follow each step in mindfulness. Breathe gently and more deeply than usual. Take hold of your breath if your mind strays.

Take a Break from Discursive Thinking

Of course we need to think. Thinking about the past and the future is essential at times so we can make wise decisions about our lives. That said, there are benefits to not always engaging in discursive thinking—that familiar experience when one thought piles upon another in a seemingly endless stream. Not only can this be exhausting, but it also keeps us from enjoying any pleasant experiences that our senses might be offering up in the present moment.

Here's an example of how discursive thinking can happen. You start to practice mindfulness of the present moment by resting your attention on what you're seeing or what you're hearing all around you. After a few minutes, you've relaxed into a pleasant feeling of calm receptiveness. But then the thought arises, "I wish I weren't sick." You could stop the thinking process right there by treating "I wish I weren't sick" as nothing more than an arising thought that will soon pass away. Instead, you embark on what I think of as the equivalent of a guitar riff. You take that simple "theme"—"I wish I weren't sick"—and the riff begins: "I'm going to have a horrible day"; "I may never feel well again"; "My life is going from bad to worse." Soon that initial thought has mushroomed into a series of thoughts that contain every stressful scenario you can come up with. It's taken you away from the relaxing practice of simply being mindful of what you're seeing or hearing in the world around you. In fact, it's colored everything about your day and left you feeling miserable.

No one can empty the mind of thoughts altogether, but with practice, when a thought such as "I wish I weren't sick" arises, you can learn to simply acknowledge its presence and then let it pass out of your mind the same way the sound of a bird singing arises in your awareness and then is gone. Taking a break from discursive thinking by resting your attention on what's going on around you puts you in touch with the present moment. It's also calming and restorative. In the words of Ayya Khema from her book *Being Nobody, Going Nowhere*:

> If we didn't give the body a rest at night, it wouldn't function very long. . . . The only time the mind can have

The Present Moment as a Refuge 127

a real rest is when it stops thinking and starts only experiencing. . . . Once verbalization stops for a moment, not only is there quiet but there is a feeling of contentment. . . . That quiet, peaceful space is the mind's home. It can go home and relax just as we do after a day's work when we relax the body in an easy chair.

The next two practices provide further help for learning to curb the constant stream of thoughts in the mind.

Three-Breath Practice

I adapted this from a practice that Tony devised to teach mindfulness at Folsom Prison, where he's a volunteer chaplain. He calls it the "three-breath trip." It's been tremendously helpful to the inmates, especially because they live in an environment that's not conducive to formal meditation.

Here's how it works. Whatever you're doing at any moment, switch your attention to the physical sensation of three in-breaths and three out-breaths. That's all there is to it. It's a simple but powerful practice—and only takes a few seconds.

Three-breath practice grounds you in your body, which brings your attention to what's going on right now in your life, because your body is always in the present moment. Most of us spend a lot of time unaware that we're lost in thoughts—often stressful and judgmental ones. They may be about the past or about the future, or they may even be a running commentary on our present-moment experience. Three-breath practice brings you into the present moment and, by doing so, provides healing relief from all that mental chatter. Because I don't seem to be able to control the scenarios my mind cooks up whenever it pleases, some days it feels as if three-breath practice is the only thing that keeps me sane!

One afternoon, during the time I was working on the revised edition of this book, I lay down for my daily nap—a necessity with my illness. But instead of being able to relax my mind and body, my mind started churning with a half dozen ideas for new material I wanted to include in the book. Then I started worrying that I'd forget these new ideas. And so I gave in, grabbed a pad of paper and a pen, and took a few notes. Then I returned to the task at hand—that nap—but my mile-a-minute thinking resumed. It was anything but restful.

I could feel the tension escalating in both my mind and my body because I badly needed to nap. So I tried three-breath practice. I took three conscious breaths by paying attention to the physical sensation of the breath as it came in and went out of my body. In that short space of time, all that mental activity—which was exhausting physically, too—gave way to a sense of ease. Then I said to myself, "It's time to nap," and I was able to. I'd only add to these instructions: "Repeat as necessary!"

I use this practice several times a day. I like doing it at random; no matter what I'm engaged in, I'll stop long enough to take three conscious in-breaths and out-breaths. As a bonus, when I exhale on that third breath, a feeling of peaceful calm comes over me, sometimes strong, sometimes slight—I'll take either one.

Three-breath practice is beneficial in a second way. When you find yourself in a difficult or antagonistic situation where you might react impulsively and later regret it, intentionally switching your attention to three conscious breaths gives you the time and space to reflect before speaking or acting. This makes it much more likely that you'll react in a skillful way to whatever situation you're facing.

Drop-It Practice

I devised this practice one day when I was particularly fed up by my constant worrying about the effects of chronic illness on my future. To try it, start by learning a simple exercise. First, consciously take your mind *out* of the present moment and into the past by remembering something you blame yourself for, something you regret, or something that simply makes you sad. For me, the sad memory might be of the profession I gave up or of the missed birthday parties for my two granddaughters. Also, there are treatments I regret having tried, and recalling them gives rise to stressful thoughts such as "Am I sicker today because of that potentially toxic antiviral I took for a year with no positive results?" For a caregiver, the memory might be of a trip that had to be canceled because your loved one was too sick to go.

Now, keep this sad or stressful memory strong in your mind and then . . . *drop it.* As you do this, immediately direct your attention to some current sensory input. It could be something you see or hear or smell. It could be the feel of your feet on the ground or the sensation of the breath coming in and going out of your body. Can you feel the relief?

If not, try the exercise again. After a few repetitions, you'll find that at the command, "Drop it," the stressful memory is gone and so is the suffering that accompanied it. With your mind in the present moment, maybe you hear a bird chirping or feel the sensation of a breeze on your body or see a beautiful print on the wall or smell something cooking in the kitchen. As Thich Nhat Hanh says in the epigraph that heads this chapter, "When we settle into the present moment, we can see beauties and wonders right before our eyes." If you're not having success with this exercise, try it while keeping your eyes closed as you focus on the memory. Then, as you drop it, open your eyes and pay attention to whatever sensory input is there in the present moment.

Now let's move to part two of the exercise. Consciously take your mind out of the present moment by thinking of something in the *future* that you're worried about or that's a source of stress or agitation for you. It could be something personal or it could be thoughts about the future of the world. I have a recurring thought that is a tremendous source of stress—it's the fear that Tony will get ill or have an accident and will need me at his side in the hospital to deal with doctors and to care for him, which I won't be able to do.

Whatever unpleasant thought you've brought to mind about the future, as you did in the first part of the exercise, keep this thought strong in your mind and then . . . *drop it.* Again, immediately direct your attention to what's going on right around you at this moment—a sight, a sound, a physical sensation.

In a nutshell, that's the exercise:

Take your mind back in time to a stressful memory, and drop it.

Take your mind forward in time to a stressful thought, and drop it.

When you drop it, you relax into the present moment and the suffering that was generated by your thoughts lifts as if you've shed a heavy weight.

Once you've learned this as an exercise, you can turn it into a mindfulness practice without consciously bringing to mind a stressful thought about the past or the future. Here's how. Whenever you realize that you're ruminating about the past or worrying about the future, say to yourself, "Drop it." And there you'll be, in the present moment. As with three-breath practice, even if that moment is accompanied by bodily discomfort, it will be easier to relax into the discomfort, riding it like a wave, because you won't be making it worse by adding to it the mental suffering that comes with stressful thoughts. I know my mind will wander into that past- and future-suffering territory again and again, but I also know that I can bring it back to the present moment with a simple "drop it" instruction.

Drop-it practice was tremendously helpful to me a few years ago when I was nervous about an appointment with my surgical oncologist to discuss the results of a breast MRI I'd had a few days before. This was my first MRI since the surgery I'd had to remove the lump in my breast.

To get to the appointment, I had to do something unusual for me: drive forty minutes on the freeway by myself, because Tony (who usually drives me) was out of town. There I was, driving sixty-five miles per hour on a freeway packed with cars, but my mind was elsewhere, worrying about the test results. I was busy mocking up one worst-case scenario after another. Then I remembered a quote from Thich Nhat Hanh: "If we practice mindfulness, we always have a place to go when we're afraid."

Inspired, I gently but firmly said, "Drop it." Then I turned my attention to the present moment. The first thing I noticed was that I was moving *really* fast. I told myself to try to stay in the moment by experiencing what it was like to be driving a car on a freeway. And what an experience it was. I felt as if I were on the Autopia ride at Disneyland. It was quite a feat to stay exactly between the painted lines while driving so fast. I was impressed with my skills! And I was amazed at how dozens of cars right around me were going just as fast but not crashing into each other. It occurred to me that this was an exquisite example of social order at work. I enjoyed every minute of the drive. And that MRI result? It was normal.

Here's a second example of when I used this practice. In retrospect, it was a situation that was quite mundane. Recall when I broke my ankle right after Tony left for a month-long retreat. The ankle healed, but I was left with an uncomfortable swelling and tingling in the ball of my foot and in my toes. My primary doctor referred me to a podiatrist. I thought, "What a treat—a doctor's visit that has nothing to do with my illness!" Tony had a conflicting obligation, so I drove myself to the two thirty appointment.

By three o'clock I was on the examining-room chair, my mind spinning with a list of grievances about the past thirty minutes and with anticipatory irritation about the future. First, the person who'd scheduled the appointment gave me faulty directions to the office, so I drove in circles for ten minutes, worried that I'd be late. Second, once I found the place, I had to sit in the waiting room for more than twenty minutes. Third, the person who showed me to the examining room said the doctor was currently seeing a patient and had one other person ahead of me. Fourth, the special podiatry examining chair appeared to be designed for my discomfort.

Angry about the past thirty minutes, irritated about the future (just how long *would* it be until the doctor came in?), I closed my eyes and silently said, "Drop it." In the space created by those two words, the thought arose that I knew nothing about the room in which I was sitting. What color were the walls? Did the room have the same kind of false ceiling that I came to know so well as I lay on the couch in my law school office? What tools of the podiatrist's were in view? Was there a window? Was there a picture on the wall? I'd been in this room for ten minutes and couldn't answer one of those questions.

And so I opened my eyes and I began a mindful investigation of the room. As I was doing this, I noticed that my anger and irritation were gone. In fact, the exploration was so absorbing that when the doctor came in, it felt too soon because I was in the middle of examining the details of the collage on the wall. This is an added bonus of drop-it practice: it can turn an unpleasant experience into a pleasant one!

I think of moments of mindfulness, no matter how short, as moments of liberation. I've discovered that truly being present for my experience brings with it a feeling of contentment that's often tinged with awe, as I pause and take in the wonder and mystery of being alive at this moment.

Recently, one of our town's most treasured citizens passed away after a good long life. The obituary in our local paper noted that Martha loved to say, "The past is history. The future is a mystery. The present is a gift."

I hope you'll take refuge in this gift.

14

Wise Action

WHAT TO DO AND WHAT NOT TO DO

Today, like every other day, we wake up empty
and frightened. Don't open the door to the study
and begin reading. Take down a musical instrument.
Let the beauty we love be what we do.
There are a hundred ways to kneel and kiss the ground.

—RUMI

IN TEACHING US how to alleviate or put an end to the suffering in the mind, the Buddha presented the Eightfold Path, which I briefly described earlier. This chapter explores one of the practices on that path: wise action, which has a lot to teach the chronically ill and their caregivers about how to take care of themselves. Simply stated, actions that lead to the cessation of suffering are to be cultivated and actions that enhance or amplify suffering are to be avoided. *Wise inaction* can thus be thought of as simply not engaging in those actions that make our condition worse.

Since becoming sick, I've learned how crucial—yet difficult—it is to practice wise inaction, that is, to avoid actions that intensify my symptoms. Worsening symptoms give rise to both physical *and* mental suffering—sometimes so severe that I break down in sobs of despair. Dukkha in abundance—a total meltdown. This used to happen frequently, but now it's a rare occurrence, thankfully. A meltdown is not only hard on Tony but also leaves me feeling sicker.

Obviously those of us who are housebound must forgo activities that take us away from our dwelling place. I'm physically able to leave the house, but I've learned that the exacerbation of symptoms that results is seldom worth the journey. For example, a few years ago, when Tony was out of town, I discovered that the front door wouldn't open, either from the inside or the outside. The doorknob turned, but it no longer pulled the latch out of the door frame. The problem had an easy solution—install a new doorknob, something I *can* do. But I was feeling particularly sick that day; I knew that going to the hardware store to buy a doorknob would inflame my symptoms. And so I went front-doorless for a day.

Wise inaction is a challenge because I'm still working to overcome a lifetime of conditioning that led me to believe it was essential to my family's quality of life for the house to always look its best, from making sure the windows were washed to keeping the yard and walkways leaf-free in autumn. Suddenly and unexpectedly, these became actions that exacerbated my symptoms—or that I simply didn't have the energy to do in the first place. It takes tremendous discipline to avoid overexertion, even within the confines of the house and yard. I fear that my house is slowly becoming a fixer-upper. I'm trying to accept this with as much grace as possible. I keep a haiku by the eighteenth-century poet Kobayashi Issa posted in the kitchen. It's about nonharming, but I use it as a reminder to let go.

Don't worry spiders,
I keep house
casually.

Recently, I discovered a positive side to wise inaction in the form of a practice I call "doing nothing." Many years ago I heard a story about a college student in Japan who went to a Zen monk and told him that she wanted to meditate but was under too much stress to do it.

The monk said to her, "Don't meditate. Just sit and do nothing."

I never forgot this story, and a few months ago I decided to turn it into a practice. Whether this is what the monk had in mind, I can't say, but it works for me. Once or twice a day I stop whatever I'm doing and do nothing for five to ten minutes. I'm usually lying down, but sometimes I'm sitting. It can also be done standing.

Most of us never learn to do nothing. Part of the reason is that our culture doesn't value it. I've discovered that when I'm doing nothing I feel calm and receptive. Whatever arises at the sense doors, I simply receive it in a relaxed nonreactive manner. And so sounds come and go, sights come and go, physical sensations come and go (or at least change), thoughts come and go, the dog comes and goes.

Once in a while, thoughts start piling upon thoughts (that discursive thinking from the previous chapter) and I start to get lost in some well-worn narrative about my life. As soon as I become aware that this is happening, I remind myself that right now I'm *doing nothing.* Usually the thoughts take the hint and make a hasty exit. If they don't, I treat them as meaningless chatter in the mind.

This practice is relaxing, restorative, and feels good. I hope you'll try it.

Finding the Middle Ground

Can we live a good and fulfilling life when our activities are so severely curtailed? Can we act to reduce suffering, even though chronic illness has imposed limitations on us?

I've discovered that wise action lies in finding the middle ground between what we used to be able to do and the alternative of giving up on almost all activity out of fear of worsening our symptoms or out of anger over our perceived misfortune. The challenge is to find the balance between too much and too little.

In *A Still Forest Pool*, Ajahn Chah talks about his teaching method. I use his discourse as a guide for determining what is wise action, given my limitations:

> It's as though I see people walking down a road I know well. To them the way may be unclear. I look up and see someone about to fall into a ditch on the right-hand side of the road, so I call out to him, "Go left, go left!" Similarly, if I see another person about to fall into a ditch on the left, I call out, "Go right, go right!" That is the extent of my teaching. Whatever extreme you get attached to, I say, "Let go of that too." Let go to the left, let go to the right. Come back to the center, and you will arrive at the true Dharma.

The key to wise action for the chronically ill, then, is to avoid extremes. If we veer too far to the one side and act as if we have the stamina and physical abilities we used to have, we risk overexertion that could land us in bed for days. But if we veer too far to the other side and avoid all activities and all contact with people, we risk missing out on experiences that can give us an emotional lift; even worse, we risk falling into despair. Either extreme increases our suffering (and that of our caregivers) and so is not wise action. The challenge is to find that middle ground.

One Thing at a Time

A valuable guideline for wise action comes from the Korean Zen master Seung Sahn: "When reading, only read. When eating, only eat. When thinking, only think."

I look upon this as a caution about multitasking. Doing one thing at a time is particularly good advice for the chronically ill whose symptoms are exacerbated if there's too much sensory input. It takes discipline to break our ingrained habit of multitasking. Mindfulness practice helps because, unless we consciously pay attention to the present moment, we can find ourselves engaged in multiple tasks without even realizing it.

One day in July 2015, I put my relationship to multitasking to the ultimate test . . . and failed miserably. Innocently enough, I turned on my TV to watch a tennis match I'd recorded of Serena Williams playing at Wimbledon. Tennis fans everywhere were keeping track of Serena's matches at Wimbledon because, if she won the tournament, she'd have the distinction of holding all four major titles at the same time, a significant achievement in the tennis world.

No one thought Serena's opponent had a chance against her, that is until the young Brit, Heather Watson, won the second set and was ahead in the third—and deciding—set. Suddenly this was the match to watch. It's the kind of thrilling match we tennis fans wait for. I don't even care who wins. I just like the excitement of a close and well-played match.

This was the perfect setup for me to have a good time.

But I didn't. Why? Well, I had an article I'd been working on for several weeks. Even though there was no deadline for me to finish it, and even though I'd turned on the TV specifically to watch this match, I picked up a hard copy of the piece and started editing it. When I finished an editing pass—with the TV still on—I entered my written changes into my computer, printed the piece out again, and made another editing pass.

Of course, unless one possesses superpowers, it's impossible to simultaneously be looking at the TV *and* the work in front of you. So what did I do? It's embarrassing to admit, but here goes.

As I edited, I listened to the TV commentators call the match. When I heard them shout "Spectacular shot!" or "How did she ever get to that ball?" or "Unbelievable point!" I rewound the recorder and then watched the play they had been so excited about.

Then I'd let the match continue while I looked back down at my work, struggling both to find my place in the article and to switch my focus back to the subject I was writing about. And, of course, the next time I heard something such as "What a point!" . . . I'd do the same thing.

Here's a summary of my experience:

I did not enjoy the tennis match. I was never able to get into the flow of the match or into the emotional intensity that both players were feeling. In addition, when I rewound to watch those spectacular points, I missed the fun of being surprised, because I knew what was about to happen.

I did not enjoy the writing. Just as it was hard to get into the flow of the tennis match, it was hard to get into the flow of the writing because, as soon as I'd focus on the content of the piece, I'd have to stop, rewind the recorder so I could watch the "spectacular" point, and then try to find the place on the hard copy where I'd left off. I didn't enjoy it and, what's more, it was mentally exhausting.

It took me twice as long to watch the tennis match. Because of all this pausing and rewinding, it took a long time to get through the match. It's hard enough with my illness to watch tennis at all (trying to follow the back-and-forth of the ball can be fatiguing); now my little "stop and rewind" routine had dragged the match out for hours.

I was irritated and cranky. The tennis kept interrupting my writing and the writing kept me from enjoying the tennis. I'd done a great job of making myself miserable!

I was (to use our household word for it) trashed afterward. When I tried to take my midday nap, my physical symptoms had been so inflamed by this crazy multitasking scheme that I wasn't able to get my body to calm down and rest; as a result, I felt awful the remainder of that day and the next one, too.

This experience convinced me more than ever that multitasking rarely mixes well with chronic pain and illness. Sure, some multitasking works fine: eating a snack while reading or watching TV. But when activities require concentration in order to do them well or even enjoy them, I've resolved anew: *one thing at a time.*

Pacing

Pacing refers to alternating periods of activity and rest. The idea is to stay within the limits of what our health can handle so as not to exacerbate our symptoms.

Pacing is the perfect example of combining wise action and wise inaction to improve quality of life for the chronically ill. It's the single best "treatment" I've found, so it's sad that I'm still struggling to master this skill. First, I have a love-hate relationship with it. On the one hand, I love pacing because it decreases the chances that my symptoms will flare. On the other hand, I hate it because it keeps me from doing everything I want to do.

Second, I'm much better at pacing when I'm at my best, as opposed to when I'm at my worst. I raise this because failing at pacing is generally considered to be the result of overdoing things when you're feeling *good* and then paying for it later, often by being confined to bed for a time. This is called the "push-crash cycle." I can do that too, but in this complicated relationship I have with pacing, I'm more likely to fail at it by overdoing things when I'm already feeling lousy. I call this the "crash-crash cycle." I've learned I'm not alone in doing this.

The reason that some of us tend to ignore pacing when we're feeling particularly sick or in pain is because being active distracts us from our symptoms; it keeps us from tuning in to how our bodies feel. Of course, eventually, the time comes when our minds take charge and say, "That is *enough* for now." Then we give in and rest, but we also have to live with feeling worse due to all that extra activity.

I hope you'll give pacing a try. We can work on it together. Here are four suggestions that can help you succeed with this "treatment":

Make a schedule. Create a schedule for the day that incorporates rest in between each activity you want or have to do, be it mental or physical. This way you're dividing your activities into manageable chunks of time. Simply having that schedule in front of you will keep you from deviating from it too much. Without set time frames, you're likely to lose track of time and keep at an activity much too long. Some people find it helpful to set a timer; when it goes off, they know it's time to stop whatever they're doing and rest for a while.

Do tasks more slowly. Many of us tend to do things quickly. Slowing down is an excellent way to pace. When you catch yourself going faster and faster—perhaps folding the laundry or doing the dishes—consciously tell yourself to slow down. Not only will you save energy but you're also more likely to enjoy the task.

Try the 50 percent rule. Decide what you can comfortably do on a given day and then only do 50 percent of it. This is a great pacing strategy because most of us overestimate what we can comfortably do, so the 50 percent rule keeps us safely within our limits. I recommend thinking of that unexpended 50 percent as a gift you're giving yourself to help you ease the difficulties of living with chronic pain and illness.

Use three-breath practice to stop yourself when you're doing too much. When you suspect that you're overdoing it and ignoring your body's signals to rest, stop and take three conscious breaths as described in the previous chapter. This switches your attention to your body and enables you to realize that you've been doing too much as a way of distracting yourself from unpleasant physical sensations. With this in mind, try reflecting with self-compassion on those sensations: "This is what pain feels like"; "This is what sickness feels like." Then, instead of resuming that distracting activity, focus on self-care by resting.

A final word on pacing. Expect the unexpected. No matter how carefully you've planned to pace yourself, as John Lennon sang in "Beautiful Boy," "Life is what happens to you while you're busy making other plans." When that happens, don't blame yourself for getting off course and don't abandon pacing. Instead, start where you are and try again. Remember the Korean Zen Master Ko Bong's "Try Mind"? It's a perfect companion to pacing.

Caregivers: What to Do and What Not to Do

Caregivers also find themselves forced to reevaluate wise action (and inaction) in light of this new and unexpected change in their lives. Whether you are the spouse, partner, child, or parent of a chronically ill person, activities away from home that were a source of joy may suddenly be severely curtailed because you have to stay home to help the person in your care. Even at home, your ability to interact and socialize with your loved one may be severely limited by his or her illness. In addition, you may feel overwhelmed by your new responsibilities—both extra physical tasks and the need to provide a new kind of emotional support for the person under your care.

Under the category of wise inaction, don't try to be Super Caregiver by forcing yourself to do every single thing you can for your loved one—and always with 100 percent enthusiasm. If you do that, you may burn out fast, and that won't benefit either one of

144 *Turnarounds and Transformations*

you. So pace yourself, just like the person in your care should be doing. Schedule time for *caregiver inaction*, if I may call it that. This could mean going out to lunch with a friend or, if your caregiver duties keep you at home, doing something enjoyable for yourself. I *want* Tony to take time for caregiver inaction. I think of it as one way I can show my appreciation for everything he does for me.

Under the category of wise action, I have four suggestions:

Share with a friend or family member how hard it is for you at times. Confiding in someone who can offer you the kind of emotional support that you're giving to the person in your care eases your own burden. If you don't have anyone you can lean on in this way, you'll find at least a dozen online support groups that are just for caregivers. You might look into these groups even if you have someone in person to talk to, because connecting with other people who share your circumstances can make a tremendous difference in your quality of life. Not only will you realize you're not alone, but you'll also feel *understood*. In addition, you can help each other problem solve when specific issues arise.

Treat yourself with compassion over this unexpected change in your life. There will be days when you're not up to the task of caregiving; you may even be resentful. Instead of feeling guilty and judging yourself negatively for what is a natural response to have at times, use one of the self-compassion practices from chapter 8. Now *that* would be wise action!

Remember that just because you can't cure your loved one doesn't mean you can't do things that will help him or her feel better. This could mean playing a board game, reading aloud to him or her, or offering a massage. After I'd been sick for a while, I noticed a change in what Tony was delivering to me in bed each night for dinner. All of a sudden, I was receiving a gourmet meal that he'd taken great care to prepare. I didn't ask him, but I suspect he realized he couldn't cure this illness (over a dozen doctors couldn't, so how could he?), but cooking a delicious meal was something he *could* do to improve my quality of life. And I think it lifts his spirits, too. That meal has become the highlight of my day. I wish with all my heart that everyone had the support I have.

Take care of your own health. The best way to assure that you can give your loved one the care you want him or her to have is to take positive steps to protect your own health—both your physical and your mental health.

15

Zen Helps

Everything
Just as it is,
as it is,
as is.
Flowers in bloom.
Nothing to add.
—ROBERT AITKEN

ALTHOUGH I'M NOT a student of Zen Buddhism, I love to read the teachings and commentaries of Zen masters. I'd like to describe three ways in which Zen has helped me live well with chronic illness. Each of these has formed itself into a practice for me.

First, Zen has a unique ability to shock the mind out of its conventional way of perceiving the world. I can count on Zen to give me a fresh perspective on my own thinking or to take me beyond thinking altogether. Second, Zen teachings help us realize how little we know for certain. Not only does this encourage me to question my lifelong assumptions, but it also serves as a reminder to stop engaging in that fruitless task of trying to predict what will happen next in my illness (and my life). And, oh, is it liberating to be relieved of the burden of having to know everything! Finally, Zen masters often teach by using poetic forms. As this verse from Soen Nakagawa illustrates, the poetry of Zen inspires us to see the world through new eyes:

> *All beings are flowers*
> *blossoming*
> *in a blossoming universe.*

As a bonus, the Zen way of conveying the Buddha's teachings—whether by shocking the mind, by pointing to how little we know for certain, or by using poetic language—can often set off a good old-fashioned belly laugh for me, the medicinal effects of which are well documented.

Shocking the Mind

Koans are stories or dialogues from the Zen tradition. They are great mind-shockers because they can't be understood by using conventional thinking skills. The most famous commentator on koans, Mumon (as he is called in Japanese; or in Chinese, Wu-men), said that in investigating Zen, we must "cut off the mind road." The mind road is like a groove we've worn into our consciousness. That groove consists of the endless stream of thoughts and stories we repeatedly spin that cloud our ability to experience the world with a fresh mind or, as Shunryu Suzuki famously said, a beginner's mind.

Take this koan:

> A monk asked Ummon, "What is Buddha?"
> Ummon replied, "A dried shit-stick."

Yes, a dried shit-stick. By way of explanation, I'll just say we now use toilet paper instead of sticks for this purpose. There are dozens of commentaries on this one koan. In *Two Zen Classics*, Katsuki Sekida writes this about it:

> The student asks seriously, "What is Buddha?" Perhaps he is imagining the glorious image of the Buddha pervading the whole universe. The answer comes like a blow to smash such an image. This kind of answer is called "breaking the thinking stream of consciousness."

Sekida's reference to the Buddha as a shit-stick smashing our glorious image of him cuts our mind road right off. It takes us out of our conventional way of thinking into a fresh awareness of the way things are. Because a shit-stick brings to mind something permeated with bacteria and viruses, I interpret this koan as meaning that even my diseased, aching body is a buddha, and so this body itself can be a vehicle for liberation, for freedom, for awakening. In his commentary on this koan, Robert Aitken invokes a similar image. In *The Gateless Barrier*, he recalls a poem he wrote while a prisoner in a Japanese internment camp during World War II:

> *In fermenting night soil*
> *fat white maggots*
> *steam with Buddhahood.*

Reading Aitken's poem, I think of my chronically ill, "fermenting" body, just *steaming* with Buddhahood. With images of shit-sticks and maggots, Zen shocks my mind into seeing that this diseased body can be a vehicle for awakening.

Oh, and this shit-stick koan gives me a good belly laugh!

Robert Aitken's teacher in the Zen path was Koun Yamada,

one of the great Zen masters of the twentieth century and the author of a commentary on Zen koans called *The Gateless Gate*. In his discussion of a koan called "Tozan's Sixty Blows," Yamada tells the story of the ancient Zen master Bokushi, who was known for his severe approach. If a student wasn't ready to receive the teachings, Bokushi would shove him out the door and slam it. One day, Bokushi was pushing his student Unmon out the door and Unmon's leg got caught and broke. Yamada writes:

> "Ouch!" he cried, and in that instant Unmon suddenly attained great enlightenment. Just "Ouch!," nothing else, no subject or object, neither relative nor absolute, just "Ouch!" This was Unmon's great enlightenment.

This story always inspires me. It's a vivid reminder that bringing undivided attention to the pain in our bodies or in our minds just might shock us into awakening—or at least give us a taste of it. No subject or object. Just life as it is, chronic illness and all.

Don't-Know Mind

Many Zen koans begin by posing a question:
"If you say there is no self, who is saying that?"
"Does a dog have Buddha nature?"
"What is the self?"
These koans used to frustrate me. Now I treat them as questions without answers. To put a different spin on "No self, no problem," I respond to these koans with "No answer, no problem." I used to react with anxiety and with anger to the question of whether I'll ever get over this mysterious illness. Now I try to treat it as a koan. "Will I get well?"—four words and a question mark, arising in the mind, with no answer. Treating it as a koan

changes my relationship to this question, which arises periodically whether I want it to or not. It allows me to hold it more lightly and wait for it to pass on through the mind.

"Will this antiviral cure me?" When I'd start a new treatment, attachment to the outcome came right along with popping the new pill. Now I try to treat the question of whether a treatment will cure or even help me as a koan—a question without an answer. The Korean Zen master Seung Sahn called this keeping a "Don't-Know Mind."

Don't-Know Mind is a major survival tool for me. During that period of several sleepless nights when I began to spin stressful stories about what it would be like if I couldn't sleep ever again, I'd stop and remember Seung Sahn's Don't-Know Mind. As I approached bedtime, I'd silently say, "I don't know if I'll sleep or not, so I won't make an assumption one way or the other." That thought would calm me and soon after beginning to practice with it, I again started to sleep. I got through those difficult days by keeping a Don't-Know Mind and by using the practice described in chapter 10—consciously moving the mind from the unpleasant physical sensation that accompanies a body deprived of sleep to the cultivation of one of the sublime states.

Thich Nhat Hanh comes at this Zen view of life from a different angle. He encourages us to examine each thought or precede each action with the reflection, "Am I sure?" This is a powerful teaching since attachment to views and opinions is such a source of suffering. I discovered the value of Thich Nhat Hanh's teaching many years before becoming sick. It started in the most mundane of settings—in front of a counter at a department store along with several other people, as I waited to buy a pair of pants. The clerk looked up and said, "Who's next?" A woman on my right stepped forward. I was about to say politely, "Excuse me, but I was here first," when Thich Nhat Hanh's "Am I sure?" popped into my mind, and so I let the other woman go ahead of me. I was 99 percent sure I was first, but allowing the other woman to check out before me had the most wonderful effect. It became an act of generosity to her, not only because she'd get out of the store before I would but also because I may have saved her from the embarrassment of mistakenly thinking it was her turn to go to the register. And, of course, in the end, was I 100 percent sure I was there first? No, just 99 percent sure.

That mundane setting planted the seed for a practice that is central to my life as a chronically ill person.

"This doctor doesn't want to treat me." Am I sure? Maybe he's terribly overbooked today.

"This friend doesn't care about me anymore." Am I sure? Maybe her attention has to be focused on her family or on problems at work.

"I'll never get better." Am I sure?

"I'm not leading a productive life anymore." Am I sure?

I have used Thich Nhat Hanh's three short words hundreds of times to let go of assumptions and opinions, an act that allows the world to unfold as it will. I find this practice works particularly well in conjunction with Byron Katie's method for investigating the validity of our thoughts.

The Poetry of Zen

Zen teachings tend to be short and to the point. In addition to koans, they often take the form of *gathas* (short verses reminding us to be mindful) and haiku. The distinctive style and rhythms of these writing forms are poetic to the ear. They can be insightful, they can be soothing, and they too can make us chuckle.

Gathas help us dwell in the present moment as we engage in tasks of everyday living. In his book of gathas, *Present Moment*

Wonderful Moment, Thich Nhat Hanh says that gathas are "exercises in both meditation and poetry." Here's his gatha for washing our feet:

> *Peace and joy in each toe—*
> *my own peace and joy.*

And his gatha for throwing out the garbage:

> *In the garbage I see a rose.*
> *In the rose, I see the garbage.*
> *Everything is in transformation.*
> *Even permanence is impermanent.*

In my early years of Buddhist practice, when mindfulness of the present moment was new to me, I carried this little gem of a book everywhere.

I also love a book of gathas called *The Dragon Who Never Sleeps*, by Robert Aitken. His gathas are indeed exercises in meditation and poetry. Many of them also make me laugh. Poetic mindfulness plus a laugh—great medicine for the chronically ill.

Here's a sampling of Aitken's gathas:

> *When wayward thoughts are persistent*
> *I vow with all beings*
> *To imagine that even the Buddha*
> *Had silly ideas sometimes.*

> *When traffic is bumper to bumper*
> *I vow with all beings*
> *To move when the world starts moving*
> *and rest when it pauses again.*

Raking the leaves from my yard
I vow with all beings
To compost extraneous thoughts
And cultivate beans of the Tao.

Haiku is a form of Japanese poetry that follows a set structure. They are a favorite form of expression for Zen masters and Zen students. My favorite haiku master is the eighteenth-century poet Kobayashi Issa. He lost his mother at the tender age of two and lost three of his own children when they were infants. And yet the haiku he wrote—especially about little creatures—never fail to make me smile:

Climb Mount Fuji,
O snail,
but slowly, slowly.

Mosquito at my ear,
does it think
I'm deaf?

I'm going out,
flies, so relax—
make love.

I am so moved by how this man, whose life was filled with personal tragedy, could write poems of such careful observation, of such creativity, and often of such unbridled joy. I'll close with a haiku from Issa that illustrates all three ways in which "Zen helps":

The world of dew
is the world of dew
And yet, and yet . . .

Issa's poetic use of words enables me to see the world through new eyes—eyes that keep a Don't-Know Mind. "Dew is dew," he appears to assert, but the last line of the haiku tells me that nothing is certain. The fleeting nature of dew is such that almost as soon as we see it, it changes into something else. Finally, the last line of the haiku shocks me out of the mind groove that's worn into my consciousness—that groove of the seemingly fixed identity: sick person. And so I could change Issa's words to:

A sick person
is a sick person
And yet, and yet . . .

Yes, Zen helps.

Balancing Community and Isolation

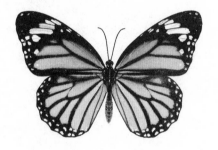

16

Communicating with Care

Take care not to:
talk too much
talk too fast
speak grandly of enlightenment
speak in an obnoxious manner
yell at children
ignore the people to whom you are speaking
speak of things of which you have no knowledge
—RYOKAN, FROM "MY PRECEPTS"

EVEN THOUGH BEING chronically ill means spending a lot of time alone—which is the subject of the next chapter—those of us who struggle with our health still communicate with others, just like everyone else. And many of the actions that cause the greatest suffering or bring about the greatest benefit in our lives are centered on one part of the body: the mouth. Just as the Buddha taught us that we create worlds with our mind, we also create worlds with our speech, so it is important to take great care in how we use it. For the chronically ill, speech—including letters, email, texting, and other written messages—can be supportive and nourishing or increase isolation and alienation.

According to the Buddha, wise speech is endowed with five qualities. It is truthful, spoken with good will, spoken beneficially, spoken affectionately, and spoken at the right time. These are usually shortened to three considerations: speak only when what you have to say is true, kind, and helpful.

It's hard to always be true, kind, and helpful in our speech, but we can undertake wise speech as a practice by setting the intention to keep those three qualities in mind before we open our mouths. Even the Zen poet Ryokan in the epigraph that opens this chapter precedes his list of precepts regarding speech with the gentle phrase, "Take care not to . . ." I know that, now and then, I won't speak truthfully and I'll also speak unkindly or in an unhelpful manner. But because I've set the intention to practice wise speech, as opposed to making it a pass/fail commandment, I can forgive myself when I come up short. Then I can consider how I might communicate more skillfully—and start anew. *Practice* is the operative word. With practice, we can make it a habit to put our words through the filter of true, kind, and helpful before we speak out loud—or click Send.

I've found that it's often easy to meet two of the criteria, but not all three. For example, it may be true that a friend of yours hasn't been in touch for a month, but would it be helpful to confront him or her about it? Before sending a "Why haven't you been in touch?" email, if you replace the intention to confront with the intention to inquire ("How are you doing?"), the communication might become kind and helpful. You may discover that the friend hasn't been in touch because he or she is having work or family problems, and this information gives you the opportunity to respond with compassion and support rather than focusing on your own desires and disappointments.

After becoming chronically ill, I faced an unexpected challenge in practicing wise speech. I assumed that anyone who cared about me would want to know, in detail, everything about the illness and my attempted treatments. For the first five years, after every appointment with a new specialist or after starting a new treatment, I'd write a long, detailed email, which I would then send to Jamal and Mara and a friend or two. In response, I'd typically get a few supportive sentences.

Not only did I assume that those to whom I was closest wanted to know every detail about my illness, but I now believe that I was also trying to make sure they realized just how sick I was. These detailed descriptions passed the Buddha's test of truthfulness, but in sending them out, I wasn't stopping to reflect on whether they were kind and helpful to those receiving them. Yes, I was sick, but everyone's life has its share of unpleasant experiences—they're right in that list from the first noble truth—and I wasn't speaking wisely when I failed to consider this. If Jamal was in the midst of a painful lower back flare or if Mara was overly busy with the many activities she juggles each day, surely it's neither kind nor helpful to ask them to read and respond in kind to a two-page email that's loaded with medical jargon and a detailed account of my symptoms. I was chronically ill for five years before it dawned on me that I needed to reevaluate whether I was communicating with care in regard to my illness.

When I looked more deeply, I saw that my relationship with family and friends would be richer and more enjoyable for all of us if I didn't always talk about my health. Included in the notion of wise speech is what the Buddha called noble silence—knowing when *not* to speak. So not only did I stop describing my experience with every new specialist and every new treatment, but I also looked for things to talk about with family and friends that would bring interest and joy to our relationships. Now I'm much more likely to ask about their lives instead of talking about my illness.

One time, for example, when I had a cold—"sick upon sick" I call it—I phoned Jamal on a Sunday to say hello. I opened my mouth with the intention to tell him about the cold but caught myself and, instead, asked him what he was up to. We chatted for a half-hour and I never mentioned the cold. I hung up, feeling great about our conversation. It had lifted my spirits and I hope it lifted his.

I no longer even share with Tony the details of every treatment—those to alleviate symptoms, or to help me sleep, or for the long-shot cure. I decided that I didn't want my relationship with him to be only about the illness. He's exposed to it every day as it is. Even when he's out of town, he checks in with me regularly. If I sat him down each day to analyze my symptoms, he'd listen. But unless I need feedback or advice, sharing with Tony the details of every symptom and response to a treatment would be neither kind nor helpful, even though it would meet the truthfulness test.

Noble silence doesn't spare Tony from listening during my moments of greater need—the occasional two A.M. sob-soaked outpouring of frustration or the two P.M. poor-me rant as I complain about things I can no longer do. Tony never fails to comfort me when these meltdowns occur. He's the most unselfish person I know.

When it comes to communicating with others, the chronically ill have to find a good balance. On the one hand, if we share with friends and family every detail of our illness, including any treatment we're trying or have tried, they may be overwhelmed. On the other hand, not talking to them means we're not sharing a major part of our lives. This increases our sense of isolation, and that doesn't feel good. Not a day goes by without this illness impacting my life in some way. Being able to talk to friends or

162   *Balancing Community and Isolation*

family members about it brings me closer to them. That said, I don't want to overwhelm them, because I know they have problems of their own. This need to keep assessing what to share and what not to share with others can be exhausting. No wonder I mentioned in an earlier chapter that being chronically ill can feel like a full-time job!

Chatting

In one source, when asked what constitutes wise speech, the Buddha said to practice abstaining from lying, divisive speech, abusive speech, and idle chatter. The first three are obvious, but the last one is more problematic. The Buddha cautioned against idle chatter, not only because it often includes vicious gossip but also because idle chatter—frivolous and meaningless speech—is a distraction from truly important matters such as cultivating compassion and mindfulness. In addition, engaging in frivolous talk, even innocent gossip, can give rise to envy and other mental states that are a source of suffering. Having acknowledged the pitfalls of idle chatter, now I must confess: since becoming chronically ill, it's the very type of speech I miss the most. Sometimes I long to feel healthy enough to spend the evening idly chatting away, exchanging trivial anecdotes with family and friends. Chatting can be a way to share a warm exchange, and it can lighten the burden of always focusing on serious matters.

I'm sure that caregivers also wish they had the luxury to idly chat with others more often. Tony and I live in a small town where he was once an elected official. It's hard for him to go anywhere without encountering someone he knows. For example, he frequently runs into people as he's walking down the aisles of the grocery store. They immediately ask, "How is Toni?" He's not going to lie and tell them I'm better, so inevitably he says, "She's

Communicating with Care   163

about the same." He tells me that this calculated-to-be-as-short-as-possible response is a conversation killer no matter how light-heartedly he says it. There are lots of grocery aisle topics—idle chatter though they may be—that would be fun for him to engage in: local politics, what our respective children are doing, even the weather! But my ongoing illness is the elephant in the aisle, and it's hard to get around the beast.

No doubt other caregivers face this dilemma. Tony and I have talked about how he can work around it. He's tried being the one to initiate the conversation by quickly asking how the other person is doing. (He reports mixed success.) And, as soon as he's said, "She's about the same," he's tried moving to a subject that's topical and has nothing to do with our respective families. (He reports better success.)

Dividing and Abusing

Idly chatting about how your family is doing or your plans for the upcoming week is usually at worst neutral, but I think a key concern the Buddha had about idle chatter was that it can easily degrade into divisive and abusive speech. Not only can this type of speech harm others, but it can also harm the speaker.

The antonyms for *divisive* and *abusive* are *unifying* and *cordial*, respectively. When we speak cordially to others, with the intent to bring unity to the interaction, we are being kind. In this way, wise speech goes hand in hand with our cultivation of the sublime states. In addition, we are being kind to ourselves, since divisive and abusive speech gives rise to mental states such as envy, anger, and resentment, all of which are sources of mental suffering and can worsen our physical symptoms.

If you find yourself about to speak divisively or abusively to others, a good antidote is patient endurance. Cultivating patience slows us down, making us more reflective. This enables us to check our speech before we release it into the world. (For a discussion of how to respond wisely to insensitive and hurtful comments, see chapter 9 on equanimity.)

Engaging in speech only when it is true, kind, *and* helpful is a tall order. Some days I'm relieved if I can just meet a couple of Ryokan's goals—not speaking too much or in an obnoxious manner! But then I remember that the Buddha considered wise speech to be an indispensable practice on the path to liberation and freedom. With that in mind, I redouble my effort to communicate wisely with others.

17

Connecting with Others and Appreciating Solitude

*I never found the companion
that was so companionable as solitude.*
—HENRY DAVID THOREAU

THE ISOLATION that comes from being housebound can be hard to bear. It's even harder for people who must spend most of their time in bed, or must suddenly take to bed in spite of plans to be with others. The Buddha placed a high value on being with others in community because it supports people personally as well as on the path to awakening or liberation. Readers of any faith will appreciate its value.

Before I got sick, I was active in my local community. I also co-hosted a weekly meditation group with Tony. We used a local meeting hall every Monday night. At least once a month I would lead the sitting and then give a talk. We also hosted a monthly group at our house in which we discussed Buddhist readings that Tony or I had chosen and distributed for that month. The reading materials were the starting point for a spirited and often humorous two hours of reviewing our lives since we last met. This was spiritual community at its richest for me. Tony still hosts this group at our house.

I also frequently attended daylong meditation retreats led by teachers from all around the world. And twice a year I attended a ten-day silent meditation retreat, led by many of the teachers I mention in this book. When I got sick, I could no longer participate in these activities, even though the Monday night meeting hall is three blocks away and the monthly group is a room away—although if I sit off to the side and mostly listen, I'm sometimes able to join the monthly group for an hour or so. In addition to losing this precious source of spiritual support, I had to adjust to the social isolation that goes hand and hand with the illness.

Alone and Cut Off

"It's hard to distinguish between the effects of my illness and the effects of isolation," wrote a member of an online support group for people diagnosed with an illness similar to mine. I, too, have days when the isolation feels like the illness itself. People who are housebound are not just isolated from one-on-one personal contacts; we are often isolated from nature and even from the warm feel of a friendly crowd. Our best bet to see the changing seasons is on the drive to and from doctor's appointments, but these are often stress-filled outings. Similarly, our best bet to be in a crowd is in the waiting room at the doctor's office—not the most comfortable or uplifting of settings. I remember reading a blog entry from a woman with ME/CFS in which she said she went to get a blood test a week early just to be around people.

The subject of friendships can be a painful one for the chronically ill. The sudden lack of day-to-day socializing was the hardest adjustment I had to make—even harder than losing my career. It felt as if there were a hole in my heart that was once filled with the sight and sounds of other people. This chapter was the last one I wrote because I was avoiding the difficult task of putting into words the pain of coming to terms with the loss of so many friends. On an Internet site for the chronically ill, one person put it this way: "Friends slipped away slowly." Another said, "All my friends have gone missing."

As I was preparing this book, I was looking through the contents of a folder and came across a note I wrote in June 2002. It caught my attention because, since becoming sick, I've read about other people having written similar notes to family and friends after being diagnosed with a chronic illness that is invisible to others—arthritis, lupus, cancer, diabetes, heart disease, fibromyalgia. After writing the note, I copied it, attached two essays from a book edited by Peggy Munson called *Stricken: Voices from the Hidden Epidemic of Chronic Fatigue Syndrome*, and sent the packet to four close friends:

> *I'm sorry I couldn't join all of you for lunch today as I'd planned. Unless people have known someone in my situation, it must be hard to understand why I can't do everything since I can do some things and since I seem to look fine.*
>
> *So I thought I'd share a couple of essays. One of the women is still working, one is not. Both have been diagnosed with chronic fatigue syndrome although, as with me, the doctors don't really know why they continue to be sick. Their stories are different from mine, but there are more similarities in our day-to-day experience than there are differences.*

I don't need you to do anything after reading these essays; I'll just feel better knowing you're aware of what's going on with me right now. See you soon.

Love,
Toni

None of these friends are a presence in my life now. And so it goes for many of the chronically ill. As I said earlier, Byron Katie's inquiry has helped me cope with the loss of so many friends, but I vividly remember how I felt when I so carefully composed that note in 2002. I was terrified that a lot of my friends would "go missing." And that turned out to be the case.

Chronic illness takes its toll on friendships for several reasons. We become undependable as companions, often having to cancel plans at the last minute if it turns out we can't get out of bed on the day of a scheduled commitment. Even if we can visit, it may only be for twenty minutes and that may be too short a time for people to commit to. (Their drive to see us may be longer than the time we're able to socialize.) Some people are uncomfortable being around those who are chronically ill. Some people no longer know what to talk about around us, believing that sharing stories about their activities will make us feel bad. And, living in the world of the sick, we gradually have less and less in common with those with whom we worked and played.

Knowing these reasons doesn't make the isolation any less painful an adjustment as we watch people disappear from our lives one by one, some after dozens of years of friendship. On top of this painful personal experience, we also encounter all the "healthy living" advice that warns us that maintaining an active social life enhances both mental and physical health. And so worry is added to isolation.

The Aloneness Spreads

Caregivers may also find themselves socially isolated because their loved one can't accompany them outside the house or apartment. Tony had a first taste of that lifestyle change on our trip to Paris, unaware it was to become a permanent feature of his life. "I've lost my companion out in the world," he's often said to me. The loss is more profound than not being able to go to dinner or the movies together. A lot of the sadness comes from those moments of lost intimacy, such as the cherished drive home from a party when Tony and I would have fun debriefing each other about the interactions we'd had—who we enjoyed chatting with, who we hoped to never see again.

Tony and I were fortunate to be best friends as we ventured out into the world. Now, in regard to social activities, he's housebound most of the time, too. People who would invite us over as a couple rarely invite Tony over by himself. This is a common experience for the partner of a chronically ill person. It's an odd social phenomenon since, when a person is single, couples have no hesitation including him or her in their social activities. Perhaps people think that Tony wouldn't want to come by himself or that I'd feel bad being left behind. We don't know.

Even at home, caregivers may be isolated from their loved one. Some days, my ability to visit with Tony is severely limited. This puts caregivers at a dual disadvantage. They're not just alone; they're alone with their worries and their frustration at not being able to make their loved one better.

In-Person Friendships

I do have a few friends who've told me they'd like to visit, but I only see two people regularly because that's all I can handle.

Connecting with Others and Appreciating Solitude 171

Oddly enough, neither of them were part of my life when I got sick in 2001. I mentioned my friend Dawn earlier—our children went to nursery school together, but when they were teenagers, she and I grew apart and the friendship all but dried up. I hadn't seen her for almost ten years. When she learned I was sick, she began visiting, even if only for twenty minutes—and she's kept it up. When we arrange a visit, sometimes at my house and sometimes at a local café, we proceed on the assumption that I'll be well enough to keep the date. Despite her busy life—real estate agent, wife, mother of three, grandmother of six—if I have to cancel at the last minute, she gracefully accepts the abrupt change in plans. The unpredictability of my day-to-day condition does not bother her.

The same is true of my other regular in-person visitor, Richard (you'll remember him from the broken ankle incident in chapter 4). He knows I may have to cancel at the last minute, and he simply doesn't mind. I'm fortunate; a lot of people aren't as understanding as Dawn and Richard. As a result, people who are chronically ill become gun-shy. This, of course, increases our isolation.

Staying Close to Family

Chronic illness also affects family relationships. I often feel isolated from my grown children's lives. I used to travel frequently to visit them, but I'm unable to do so now. As a result, I rarely see Mara and her family in person. I see Jamal and his family more often because they're only a bit more than an hour's drive away and come to visit when they can.

I depend on the digital age to help me stay close to Jamal and Mara. My principal mode of communication with them is texting (it's hard for me to talk on the phone). I lie on the bed with my laptop; they use their smartphones or their computers, and we chat back and forth. Once, when Mara and her family were visiting, she even texted me from the living room to share what was going on in the front of the house! And when my son-in-law, Brad, was graduating from UCLA's Anderson School of Management, I was lying on my bed, thinking about the graduation ceremony I was missing, when suddenly this text from Mara's phone popped up on my computer screen: "Brad's name was just called and he's walking across the stage!" It made me feel less isolated on this special day.

I treasure these interactions with Jamal and Mara. You can try any number of modern modes of communication to help you stay in touch with family—email, texting, Skype, FaceTime, social media sites. And, of course, there's still the old-fashioned telephone! Despite this dizzying array of alternatives, I still wish I could visit Jamal and Mara and their families on their home turfs. When it comes to family, nothing quite replaces being in each other's physical presence.

Cyber Relationships

When I surf the web, looking to connect with people, I find myself drifting to blogs and other sites where people are similarly sick. I've encountered bloggers who range in age from a sixteen-year-old girl with ME/CFS who can rarely leave the house, to a mom with multiple sclerosis who is struggling to raise two girls, to a man in his sixties with diabetes who writes a daily blog from his bed.

These people come from many different backgrounds and don't necessarily use Buddhist terminology as they navigate their lives—the teenager is a devoted Mormon, for instance—but they are writing about mental suffering. My spiritual community now includes these chronically ill people who have come face-to-face with the fact of suffering in their lives and who, like me, are struggling to accept it and to cultivate compassion for their own illness and for those they encounter on the Internet. The fact that they don't share Buddhism per se with me doesn't matter—they're part of my community.

It's a limited community for me because, many days, my illness prevents me from reading and answering more than an email or two and checking a few social media sites. However, many of the chronically ill aren't as limited as this. Whatever your illness, it's easy to find support groups and blogs with people who are facing the same difficulties that you are. I know from my Internet wanderings that these online contacts can be a lifeline. One woman left a comment on a blog saying she'd been overwhelmed by loneliness until she found blogs written by people who were similarly sick. She said that for the first time since becoming ill, she was able to connect with people who understood her.

Opinions abound on the pros and cons of hanging out on social media sites, such as Facebook. In my view, whether these sites enhance or diminish your quality of life depends on your situation. If you're able to go out with friends but decline so you can hang out online, that may not be a healthy choice. But if you're housebound due to physical pain or illness, or if you suffer from depression that makes it difficult to go out, online forums and private Facebook groups can be a valuable source of information and support.

I want to emphasize that the use of social media is not inherently good or bad; it's an individual choice. If it makes you feel sad to look at pictures that friends and family post of their travels or other fun activities, don't use those sites. Practice self-compassion and make the choice that's wise for you.

In addition to forming relationships on the web, I've found good company by nurturing some "email friendships." A few years ago

I became friends with a woman who lives on the opposite side of the country from me. We've developed a close friendship simply by emailing each other back and forth. I write to Jennie one day; she writes back another. When I compose an email to her, I always look at the last one she sent, so I'm sure to respond to what she wrote. We initially became friends because we've both been diagnosed with ME/CFS. Gradually we discovered that we have much more in common than a shared illness. We write to each other about everything, from mundane happenings in our lives to serious issues. It's a deep and rewarding friendship even though we've never talked on the phone. It's unlikely we'll ever meet in person, although we often close our emails with the wish that we were in the same room together, chatting over coffee or tea. I'd sure like to give Jennie a big in-person hug!

Solitude

The combination of lost friends and the inability to leave the house makes isolation a fact of life for many of us. After chronic illness set in, it took me several years to realize that isolation itself is a neutral state; it's simply the fact of being alone. In the above discussion, I added the words *painful*, *sad*, and *difficult*, because that was my experience of isolation in the early years of the illness. If isolation has also been hard for you, here are some ideas to help you alleviate this source of mental suffering. To start, consider this excerpt from Paul Tillich's *The Eternal Now*: "Language . . . has created the word 'loneliness' to express the pain of being alone. And it has created the word 'solitude' to express the glory of being alone."

I came across this quotation a few years ago and decided to examine if Tillich's words could help me change how I react to being alone. To do this, I returned to Byron Katie's technique that

Connecting with Others and Appreciating Solitude 175

I learned from Mara. If you recall, Katie was caught in a cycle of stressful thoughts about the fate of her daughter who was late coming home. By repeating to herself the one thing she knew for sure—"Woman in chair, waiting for her beloved daughter"—Katie was able to stop the mental suffering and just wait until her daughter returned.

I tried this approach as a way to examine isolation ("the fact of being alone") in the context of Tillich's insight. I realized that the very same fact of isolation—"Woman in chair, alone in the house"; "Man lying on bed, alone in the bedroom"—can be accompanied by the mental state of loneliness, or it can be accompanied by the mental state of contented solitude.

My online wanderings have revealed that while for some people, isolation results in a debilitating loneliness, for others, isolation makes possible a treasured solitude. Some people value solitude because it allows them to have more control over their lives. A woman in an online support group for the chronically ill, for example, said she loves isolation because it means that no one is making demands on her. Others value solitude because it's an essential part of their spiritual practice. Another woman from the same group said, "Solitude is refreshing to the human spirit and is practiced by all religious denominations to come to know God." Indeed, there is a centuries-old culture of solitude that many people, healthy or sick, find essential to their spiritual well-being despite our culture's emphasis on the necessity of maintaining an active social life.

If you're hurting due to being alone so much, it might help to recognize that being alone in and of itself is not a negative experience. It's a neutral state—to which we sometimes add the desire for things to be other than they are (for example, to have company). When that desire for things to be different goes unfulfilled, we experience dukkha (suffering, stress, dissatisfaction with our lives). Byron Katie's technique can help here, too. Bring yourself to the present moment by describing what you're aware of physically: "Woman/Man alone in the house." Then see if without adding the desire—that felt need—for things to be different, you're able to experience a taste of serenity in that aloneness—or maybe just relief that no one is making demands on you! If you can, you'll understand that words such as *sad* and *painful* need not necessarily accompany the fact of isolation in your life.

When I got sick in 2001, I had neither this valuable tool offered by Byron Katie nor was I aware of Paul Tillich's statement. I did manage to make the journey from the "poverty" of loneliness to the "glory" of solitude, but it took several years. At first, isolation and loneliness were synonymous for me and I suffered deeply. After the initial six months of acute illness, friends rarely came to see me, and Tony was still working full-time. Even after leaving his job, he continued to be busy with work or Buddhist-related activities or with trips out of town to see our children and our granddaughter Malia. I spent a lot of time alone—and I cried a lot.

Then one day, I was listening to an audiobook, *The Dive from Clausen's Pier,* by Ann Packer. At one point, a character said, "Lonely is a funny thing. It's almost like another person. After a while it will keep you company if you let it." And, just like that, in three short sentences, my heart and mind opened to being alone. From that day on, I've been better able to welcome isolation as a friend, and the pain of loneliness has been replaced with the good company of solitude.

Of course, I'm not always successful. Some days I rejoice in the glory of solitude. Other days I feel so lonely it brings me to tears. Some days I'm content to let the small-town life of Davis unfold without knowing, as I used to, all the details of what's going on socially and politically. Other days I'm hungry for news from outside the house. Tony is well aware of this latter tendency. One day, he ran into an old friend. We knew she'd been through a painful divorce and had been having a difficult time for a few years. To Tony's delight, she told him that she'd met a man and was happily in love. Tony told me that he said to her, "Okay, ask yourself everything that Toni would want to know about him and then tell me, so that I can tell her."

When overcome with loneliness, I use the practices I've described in this book. Starting with the Buddha's teaching in the first noble truth, I recognize that all living beings face difficulties and challenges in life. Even those who aren't sick may experience the pain of loneliness. I think of Joko Beck's teaching: This is just my life; there's nothing wrong with it even if I'm lonely at the moment. Then I might move to weather practice, reminding myself that loneliness, like everything else, is impermanent. It blew in and will blow away, perhaps replaced with the serenity of solitude. Cultivating the sublime states soothes me during these blue periods; I might craft some self-compassion phrases, such as "It's so hard to feel lonely, but it will pass and I'll be okay." Tonglen practice has been extremely helpful to me, too. I call to mind everyone who, like me, is feeling lonely. I breathe in their sadness and then I breathe out thoughts of kindness, compassion, and peace. This makes me feel a deep connection to others who are lonely, and that connection in itself makes me feel less lonely. Byron Katie's inquiry gives me the tools to examine the validity of stressful thoughts that often accompany the feeling of loneliness, such as "Nobody cares about me" and "I'll always be lonely."

These Buddhist and Buddhist-inspired practices are always waiting in the wings to help transform that neutral fact of isolation from the despair of loneliness to the serenity of solitude.

It's been hard adjusting to the loss of my spiritual community, to the loss of so many friends, and lastly, to being alone much of the time. I've largely come through that struggle, but it took time, it took effort, and it took help from a lot of people—the Buddha, his followers, a philosopher, a fiction writer, and ordinary people who have been generous enough to go online and share their experiences.

18

And in the End . . .

This very place is the Lotus Land;
This very body, the Buddha.
—HAKUIN

LIVING WELL with chronic illness is a work in progress for me. Some days I still cry out:

"I can't stand this oppressive illness one more day!"
"I don't care if stressful thinking makes my symptoms worse!"
"I don't want to hear that laughter coming from the living room!"
"I don't care if this is the *Way Things Are*; I don't want to be sick and in pain!"

When this happens, I "put my head in the lap of the Buddha," as the Dalai Lama suggests, and take refuge in one of the practices I've shared in this book. The Buddha's teachings and the practices he inspired are always waiting in the wings to see me through. The Buddha continues to inspire me because he never claimed to be anything more than a human being. In fact, the Buddha found pain just as painful as you and I do, as the Buddhist texts take great care to make clear. Consider this passage from the *Connected Discourses of the Buddha* about an instance when the Buddha was cut by a stone splinter:

> Severe pains assailed him—bodily feelings that were painful, wracking, sharp, piercing, harrowing, disagreeable. But the Buddha endured them, mindful and clearly comprehending, without becoming distressed.

I take this as a reminder that the equanimity and joy we see in the many images of him are within the reach of every one of us. I never stray far from the Buddha's list from chapter 3 of the difficulties we all face at one time or another in life. I think here, too, of Joko Beck's teaching that our life is always all right. There's nothing wrong with it even if we have terrible problems. It's just our life.

In the Buddha's time, each of his monks carried a bowl when they went into the village to collect food from lay supporters. Each day, a monk ate only what was put in the bowl, whether it was filled to the top with scrumptious goodies or contained only a few morsels. Tony uses this as a metaphor for life. We have what is put in our bowls. Tony's and my bowls contain my illness and my ongoing treatment for breast cancer. At times, this has been a great source of suffering for us. But even people whose bowls are usually filled with ambrosia have days when they are only given a few grains of rice. And although Tony's and my bowls contain my health struggles, our children and grandchildren are in there, too, along with other blessings. This is what we've been given.

Some years ago I was listening to Terry Gross's *Fresh Air* on NPR. She was interviewing country music singer and songwriter Rosanne Cash. Cash had been forced to put her career on hold for several years because she had to have brain surgery for a rare but benign condition. Gross asked her if she ever found herself asking, "Why me?"

Cash said no, that, in fact, she found herself saying, "Why *not* me?" since she had health insurance, no nine-to-five job that she might lose during her long recuperation, and a spouse who was a wonderful caregiver.

Rosanne Cash's words had a profound effect on me. Now, on a day when I start to sink into that "Why me?" mood, I think of the Buddha's list and am reminded that illness is a natural part of the human life cycle. That enables me to say, "Why *not* me?" On top of that, like Rosanne Cash, I am blessed to have health insurance and a wonderful caregiver. So why *not* me?

I have a personal Facebook page with "friends," some of whom I don't know personally because they're friends of my children. In 2009, Davis was the starting point for Lance Armstrong's first race in the United States after coming out of retirement (this was before his accomplishments were discredited). In a town as small as ours, this was a major community event. Despite it being a rainy day, our local newspaper expected big crowds to gather downtown for the noontime start of the race. People would be there whom I hadn't seen for years. Feeling frustrated, cranky, and lonely because I couldn't be part of this social gathering, but also not wanting to whine online, I posted this on my Facebook page: "Lying in bed, watching the rain." My daughter's friend Stephanie, who doesn't think of me as sick because we've never met, added this lovely comment to my post: "That sounds perfect!"

I momentarily thought, "Yeah, perfect for *you*," but then I smiled, realizing that my life is indeed perfect. There's nothing wrong with it. It's what I've been given. It's just my life.

In sickness or in health, my heartfelt wish is that you be peaceful, have ease of well-being, reach the end of suffering, and be free.

And in the End . . . 183

A Guide to Using the Practices to Help with Specific Challenges

SOME PRACTICES IN THE BOOK may resonate with you, others may not. I encourage you to try them all and stick with the ones you find helpful. And don't forget to keep a Try (and Forgiving) Mind!

Suffering due to the relentlessness of physical symptoms or from the addition of new medical problems

▸ *Take solace in the fact that you are not alone*; difficult and unpleasant experiences are present in the lives of all beings. Having been born, we are subject to change, disease, and ultimately death. It happens differently for each person. This is one of the ways it's happening to you. Recall Joko Beck's teaching: your life is always all right; there's nothing wrong with it, even if you're suffering. It's just your life. The good news from the Buddha is that no matter how much you are suffering physically, there are practices that can help alleviate your mental suffering. (See chapter 3.)

185

- *Breathe in the suffering of all those who share the symptoms you're experiencing. Breathe out whatever kindness, compassion, and peace you have to give.* Because you share this particular kind of suffering with them, the thoughts you breathe out will also be directed at yourself. (See chapter 11.)
- *Repeat the metta phrases you've settled on,* directing kindness at yourself, perhaps stroking your body as you do so. (See chapter 7.)
- *Craft phrases that directly address your suffering.* Find words that are specific to the particular difficulty you're experiencing and repeat them compassionately to yourself: "It's so hard to wake up with a headache every morning"; "It feels overwhelming to have this injury on top of my illness." Recall Thich Nhat Hanh's description of one hand naturally reaching out to the other in pain. *Cultivate patient endurance* by trying to maintain a calm state of mind while also not giving up on your search for relief from your symptoms. *Open your heart to your suffering.* (See chapter 8.)
- Try Ajahn Chah's *letting go, even just a little*—taking baby steps toward peace and equanimity each time you repeat his phrases. Work on *giving in to what's happening instead of giving up.* (See chapter 9.)
- As you experience the unpleasant physical sensations, instead of reacting with aversion, *consciously move your mind toward the sublime state of kindness, compassion, or equanimity*—directing the sublime state at yourself. You can also try moving your mind to empathetic joy—feeling happy for those who are in good health. (See chapter 10.)
- *Try weather practice.* Recognize that these physical symptoms are as unpredictable as the weather and could change at any moment. The wind blew the discomfort in and it may blow it out at any moment. If a new medical problem develops, such

as an injury, recall that no forecast of the future could have been certain no matter how many precautions you took. (See chapter 4.)

▸ *Try to keep a Don't-Know Mind*, reminding yourself that you don't know how long any particular discomfort will last. It won't last indefinitely, and you might even feel better soon. Recall the Zen practice of shocking the mind and how the power of pain could provide such focused attention that the mind is shocked into a moment of awakening. Turn to the poetry of Zen to soothe the body and to feed it the medicine of laughter. (See chapter 15.)

▸ *Use Byron Katie's inquiry to question the validity of stressful thoughts*, such as "This physical discomfort will never go away" or "I can't stand this symptom one more minute." (See chapter 12.)

▸ When a thought persists about the past or future regarding the relentlessness of symptoms ("I caused them because of what I did yesterday . . . Will they ever subside?"), *acknowledge the thought and then . . . drop it*, bringing awareness to the present moment. *Try three-breath practice* to help you come out of your stories and calmly ground you in your body. *Take a break from discursive thinking* so that one simple thought doesn't turn into a barrage of stressful ones. Try Byron Katie's practice of stating what you're doing physically *right now*: "Woman lying on bed, resting"; this will take you out of your repeating round of stressful thoughts and into the present moment. (See chapter 13.)

▸ *Be sure you don't engage in unwise action*—actions that could exacerbate symptoms (such as doing too much housework). For relief, try *doing nothing*. Work on *pacing*. (See chapter 14.)

▸ Recall Munindra-ji's words and recite, *"There is sickness here, but I am not sick."* Contemplate *"Who am I?"* to help shed

A Guide to Using the Practices to Help with Specific Challenges 187

the fixed identity of "sick person." Try *sky-gazing*. If you're in bed, try virtual sky-gazing by closing your eyes and shifting your focus from the unpleasant physical symptoms to a more spacious and open experience of body and mind as part of the energy flow of the universe. (See chapter 5.)

Blaming yourself for being sick

- *Remember that we'd never speak as harshly to others as we do to ourselves,* as Mary Grace Orr discovered. *Disidentify from your inner critic.* (See chapter 8.)
- *Breathe in the suffering of all those who blame themselves for being sick. Breathe out whatever kindness, compassion, and peace you have to give.* Because you share this particular kind of suffering with them, the thoughts that you breathe out will also be directed at yourself. (See chapter 11.)
- *Repeat the metta phrases you've settled on*, directing kindness at yourself, perhaps stroking your body as you do so. (See chapter 7.)
- When you think, "It's my fault for being sick," *acknowledge the thought and then . . . drop it*, bringing awareness to the present moment. Try *three-breath practice* to help you come out of your stories and calmly ground you in your body. *Take a break from discursive thinking* so that one simple thought doesn't turn into a barrage of stressful ones. Try Byron Katie's practice of stating what you're doing physically *right now*: "Man sitting in chair, reading a book"; this will take you out of your repeating round of stressful thoughts and into the present moment. (See chapter 13.)
- As you experience the unpleasant mental state of blame, instead of reacting with aversion and self-hatred, *consciously move your mind toward the sublime state of kindness, compassion,*

or equanimity—directing the sublime state at yourself. (See chapter 10.)

- *Recall that anything can happen at any time.* This includes chronic illness. It can strike anyone at any moment despite the best of precautions; it's nobody's fault. *Try weather practice:* Recognize that blame is a mental state as unpredictable as the weather. The wind blew this painful mood in and it may blow it out at any moment. (See chapter 4.)

- *Use Byron Katie's inquiry to question the validity of stressful thoughts,* such as "It's my fault that I got sick" or "It's my fault that I don't get better." (See chapter 12.)

- Recall Munindra-ji's words and recite, "*There is sickness here, but I am not sick.*" Contemplate "*Who am I?*" to help shed the fixed identity of "sick person." (See chapter 5.)

Receiving cursory or dismissive treatment from a doctor or other medical professional

- *Ask yourself, "Am I sure?"* before deciding that the medical professional didn't want to help you. Maybe the person you saw was overwhelmed with work that day or was experiencing personal problems. If you have a follow-up appointment, try to keep a *Don't-Know Mind* until then. (See chapter 15.)

- *Use Byron Katie's inquiry to question the validity of stressful thoughts,* such as "This doctor didn't want to treat me" or "This medical person thinks I'm not really sick." (See chapter 12.)

If you decide that this doctor or other medical professional did unfairly dismiss you

- *Recall Ajahn Chah's sayings, "If no one is there to receive it, the letter is sent back" and "Don't stand up in the line of fire."*

A Guide to Using the Practices to Help with Specific Challenges   189

Practically, this means accepting that this is the way he or she relates to you and/or your illness and it's time to move on to another doctor. Then try *letting go, even just a little*—taking baby steps toward peace and equanimity each time you repeat Ajahn Chah's phrases. Work on *giving in instead of giving up* by continuing to look for good medical care. (See chapter 9.)

- *Breathe in the suffering of all those who have been treated poorly by a doctor or other medical professional. Breathe out whatever kindness, compassion, and peace you have to give.* Because you share this particular kind of suffering with them, the thoughts you breathe out will also be directed at yourself. (See chapter 11.)

- *Try directing your metta phrases at the people who treated you poorly* (they come under the category of those who are a source of stress in your life). It can be liberating to wish others well— to befriend them in your thoughts—even though they are being insensitive to you. The odds are high that this medical person has been of help to many others. Be glad for those people. (See chapter 7.)

- *Craft phrases that directly address your suffering.* Find words specific to the particular difficulty you're experiencing and repeat them compassionately to yourself: "It hurts so much to be treated dismissively by a doctor." *Cultivate patient endurance* by trying to maintain a calm state of mind while also asserting yourself with the aspiration that better treatment will result. *Open your heart to your suffering.* (See chapter 8.)

- As you experience the unpleasant mental sensations of being treated in a dismissive manner by this medical person, instead of reacting with aversion, *consciously move your mind toward the sublime state of kindness, compassion, or equanimity*— directing the sublime state at yourself. (See chapter 10.)

- If a painful thought persists about the experience, *acknowledge the thought and then . . . drop it,* bringing awareness to the present moment. *Try three-breath practice* to help you come out of your stories and calmly ground you in your body. *Take a break from discursive thinking* so that one simple thought doesn't turn into a barrage of stressful ones. Try Byron Katie's practice of stating what you're doing physically *right now*: "Woman sitting in car after a doctor's appointment"; this will take you out of your repeating round of stressful thoughts and into the present moment. (See chapter 13.)

Suffering due to the inability to visit with people or participate in family gatherings and other social events

- *Cultivate joy for those who are able to have an active social life and attend special gatherings.* This helps alleviate any envy that might arise. By cultivating joy in the joy of your family or friends who are at a particular event, you may find that you can enjoy the event through those who are there. (See chapter 6.)
- *Use Byron Katie's inquiry to question the validity of stressful thoughts,* such as "I would have had such a wonderful time at that event" or "I can't stand to be left out of socializing." (See chapter 12.)
- *Use broken-glass practice. Reflect on how all that arises passes away* and so your ability to socialize and go to events was already broken. These changes will befall everyone at some point in life. This is how it has happened to you. Then remember to look after each moment, cherishing what you still *can* do. (See chapter 4.)
- *Craft phrases that directly address your suffering.* Find words specific to the particular activity or gathering you're suffering over and repeat them compassionately to yourself: "It's so hard

A Guide to Using the Practices to Help with Specific Challenges 191

not to be able to join the family for dinner." *Open your heart to your suffering.* (See chapter 8.)

▸ *Try looking at your disappointment the way Ajahn Jumnian would. If you were able to visit or participate, that would have been fine. You weren't, so you'll find something enjoyable to do that's within your limits.* Try Ajahn Chah's *letting go, even just a little*—taking baby steps toward peace and equanimity each time you repeat his phrases. Work on *giving in instead of giving up,* by looking for what else you might do. (See chapter 9.)

▸ *Breathe in the suffering of all those who are unable to visit with friends or attend family gatherings. Breathe out whatever kindness, compassion, and peace you have to give.* Because you share this particular kind of suffering with them, the thoughts that you breathe out will also be directed at yourself. (See chapter 11.)

▸ As you experience the unpleasant mental sensations of not being able to engage in these activities, instead of reacting with resentment and anger, *consciously move your mind toward the sublime state of kindness, compassion, or equanimity*—directing the sublime state at yourself. You can also try moving your mind to empathetic joy—feeling happy for those who are able to have an active social life. (See chapter 10.)

▸ *Try saying, "This was an activity that I was able to enjoy for X years,"* using the practice inspired by Susan Saint James (whose young son died). (See chapter 9.)

▸ *Reread the discussion about loneliness and solitude.* If it suits you, explore the Internet for alternatives to traditional face-to-face relationships and activities, whether it be finding people who are similarly sick or people with whom you share non-illness-related interests. (See chapter 17.)

Feeling ignored by family or friends

▸ *Ask yourself, "Am I sure?"* before deciding that they are consciously ignoring you. They may be busy at work or sick themselves or concerned that contacting you will exacerbate your symptoms. (See chapter 15.)

▸ *Consciously counter this painful mental state by taking the initiative to connect with those you feel are ignoring you.* It's unlikely they were intentionally ignoring you. (See chapter 8.)

▸ *Use Byron Katie's inquiry to question the validity of stressful thoughts,* such as "He or she doesn't care about me" or "My family should call more often." (See chapter 12.)

▸ *Check your own communication skills.* Have you been complaining too much about your illness or going into too much detail about doctors and treatments? Can you find other subjects to talk about—shared interests and the like? (See chapter 16.)

If you decide you really are being ignored

▸ *Take solace in the fact that you are not alone;* difficult and unpleasant experiences are present in the lives of all beings. Even people who aren't sick struggle in their relationships with family and friends. Recall Joko Beck's teaching: your life is always all right; there's nothing wrong with it, even if you're suffering. It's just your life. The good news from the Buddha is that there are practices that can help alleviate your mental suffering. (See chapter 3.)

▸ *Repeat the metta phrases you've settled on,* directing kindness at yourself. Then try directing the phrases at these people (they come under the category of those who are a source of stress in your life). It can be liberating to wish others well—to befriend them in your thoughts—even if they are being insensitive to you. (See chapter 7.)

► *Craft phrases that directly address your suffering.* Find words specific to the particular difficulty at hand and repeat them compassionately to yourself: "It hurts to be ignored by those I love." *Open your heart to your suffering.* (See chapter 8.)

► *Breathe in the suffering of all those who are being ignored by family or friends. Breathe out whatever kindness, compassion, and peace you have to give.* Because you share this particular kind of suffering with them, the thoughts that you breathe out will also be directed at yourself. (See chapter 11.)

► *Try saying, "These were relationships that I was able to enjoy for X years" or "This was a friendship that lasted for X years,"* using the practice inspired by Susan Saint James (whose young son died). (See chapter 9.)

► If a painful thought persists about lost friendships, *acknowledge the thought and then . . . drop it,* bringing awareness to the present moment. Try *three-breath practice* to help you come out of your stories and calmly ground you in your body. *Take a break from discursive thinking* so that one simple thought doesn't turn into a barrage of stressful ones. Try Byron Katie's practice of stating what you're doing physically *right now*: "Woman sitting at table, eating"; this will take you out of your repeating round of stressful thoughts and into the present moment. (See chapter 13.)

► Work on *giving in to what's happening instead of giving up* by looking to see if there are other people you can reach out to. (See chapter 9.)

► *Reread the discussion about loneliness and solitude.* If it suits you, explore the Internet for alternatives to traditional face-to-face relationships, whether it be finding people who are sim-

194   *How to Be Sick*

ilarly sick or people with whom you share non-illness-related interests. (See chapter 17.)

Suffering due to uncertainty about the future

- *Take solace in the fact that you are not alone;* difficult and unpleasant experiences are present in the lives of all beings. This includes suffering over life's uncertainty. Recall Joko Beck's teaching: your life is always all right; there's nothing wrong with it, even if you're suffering. It's just your life. The good news from the Buddha is that there are practices that can help alleviate your mental suffering. (See chapter 3.)
- *Try weather practice.* Recognize that life is as unpredictable as the weather. Predicting the future is like predicting the weather. Remember Dogen's verse—how the bitterest cold may be setting the stage for something joyful. Indeed, the future could hold a lot of sunshine. (See chapter 4.)
- *Try to keep a Don't-Know Mind,* reminding yourself that you don't know how long any particular symptom or other concern will last. It won't last indefinitely, and it might change sooner than you think. (See chapter 15.)
- If a thought about the uncertainty of the future persists, *acknowledge the thought and then . . . drop it,* bringing awareness to the present moment. *Try three-breath practice* to help you come out of your stories and calmly ground you in your body. *Take a break from discursive thinking* so that one simple thought doesn't turn into a barrage of stressful ones. Try Byron Katie's practice of stating what you're doing physically *right now*: "Man lying on bed, resting"; this will take you out of your repeating round of stressful thoughts and into the present moment. (See chapter 13.)
- *Use Byron Katie's inquiry to question the validity of stressful*

thoughts, such as "I'll never get better" or "The future only holds pain for me." (See chapter 12.)

▸ As you experience the unpleasant mental sensation of uncertainty about the future, instead of reacting with worry and fear, *consciously move your mind toward the sublime state of kindness, compassion, or equanimity*—directing the sublime state at yourself. (See chapter 10.)

Coping with the disappointment of failed treatments

▸ *Craft phrases that directly address your suffering.* Find words specific to the particular difficulty you're experiencing and repeat them compassionately to yourself: "It's so hard to be disappointed yet again." *Cultivate patient endurance* by trying to maintain a calm state of mind while also not giving up on the possibility that future treatments may help. If you're blaming yourself for the failure, remember that we'd never speak as harshly to others as we do to ourselves, as Mary Grace Orr discovered. *Disidentify from your inner critic.* (See chapter 8.)

▸ *Repeat the metta phrases you've settled on,* directing kindness at yourself to soothe you in your disappointment. (See chapter 7.)

▸ *Breathe in the suffering of all those who have been disappointed by the results of a treatment. Breathe out whatever kindness, compassion, and peace you have to give.* Because you share this particular kind of suffering with them, the thoughts you breathe out will also be directed at yourself. (See chapter 11.)

▸ When a thought about a past treatment persists ("I never should have tried it . . . I should have listened to my friend who warned me the treatment would fail"), *acknowledge the thought and then . . . drop it,* bringing awareness to the present moment. *Try three-breath practice* to help you come out of your stories and calmly ground you in your body. *Take a break from discursive thinking* so that one simple thought doesn't turn into a barrage of stressful ones. Try Byron Katie's practice of stating what you're doing physically *right now*: "Woman lying on bed, reading a book"; this will take you out of your repeating round of stressful thoughts and into the present moment. (See chapter 13.)

▸ *Try looking at your disappointment the way Ajahn Jumnian would. If the treatment worked, that would have been fine. It didn't, so that's fine, too; it isn't what your body needed.* Try Ajahn Chah's *letting go, even just a little*—taking baby steps toward peace and equanimity each time you repeat his phrases. Work on *giving in instead of giving up,* by keeping up on your medical condition so you'll know if new treatments become available. (See chapter 9.)

Handling caregiver burnout

▸ *Take solace in the fact that you are not alone;* difficult and unpleasant experiences are present in the lives of all beings. Recall Joko Beck's teaching: your life is always all right; there's nothing wrong with it, even if you're suffering due to your extra responsibilities. It's just your life. The good news from the Buddha is that there are practices that can help alleviate your mental suffering. (See chapter 3.)

▸ *Breathe in the exhaustion and frustration of all those who are shouldering the responsibility of caring for a chronically ill person. Breathe out whatever kindness, compassion, and peace you have to give.* Because you share this particular kind of suffering with them, the thoughts you breathe out will also be directed at yourself. (See chapter 11.)

▸ *Try to keep a Don't-Know Mind,* reminding yourself that you

A Guide to Using the Practices to Help with Specific Challenges 197

don't know how long your loved one will need this extra attention. He or she might even feel better soon. Turn to the poetry of Zen to soothe your exhaustion and to feed it the medicine of laughter. (See chapter 15.)

- *Open your heart to your suffering.* If you're feeling that family and friends could be helping more but aren't, take compassionate action toward yourself by taking the initiative to connect with them. Often people are just waiting to be asked to help but won't make that first contact. *Cultivate patient endurance* by trying to maintain a calm state of mind while also not giving up on the possibility that future treatments may help. If you're blaming yourself for not being a good enough caregiver, remember that we'd never speak as harshly to others as we do to ourselves, as Mary Grace Orr discovered. *Disidentify from your inner critic.* (See chapter 8.)

- *Think of activities you could engage in that might be fun and relaxing for you or for you and your loved one together.* Work on *pacing.* (See chapter 14.)

- *Look for ways to talk to others about subjects of interest that aren't related to your loved one's illness.* (See chapter 16.)

- If it suits you, *explore the Internet to see if you can find support groups or blogs written by people who are also in the role of caregiver.* (See chapter 17.)

- Work on *giving in instead of giving up*, by being sure that you're taking good care of yourself. (See chapter 9.)

- Contemplate *"Who am I?"* to help shed the fixed identity of "caregiver." (See chapter 5.)

With Gratitude

Mara Tyler—my daughter. Mara is the first person who told me I should write a book. Without her encouragement, I doubt it would have happened. She's the person I turn to when I'm struggling with being sick and Tony isn't available or I don't want to burden him. She listens and responds compassionately. I feel heard, and that allows me to pick myself up and return to the practices in this book. I'm so blessed that she's my daughter.

Jamal Bernhard—my son. Jamal takes me as I am and that relieves me of a tremendous burden. If I can visit in person, that's fine. If I can't, that's fine. If I can talk on the phone, fine. If not, we'll talk when I'm able. I can call him up, tell him I'm good for five minutes, and ask him to give me the scoop on the Super Bowl. He clocks in precisely at five minutes, we exchange *love you*s, and I hang up knowing exactly what to look for in the game. Jamal doesn't treat me like I'm sick, and that makes our relationship truly special.

Bridgett Lawhorn Bernhard—my daughter-in-law. I can always count on Bridgett to be a compassionate presence for me when

I feel the need to unload about being sick all the time. It means so much to me. I also love what a conscientious parent she is. And chatting with her is such a pleasure; she always makes me laugh. Since I became chronically ill, she has become a close and treasured friend.

Brad Tyler—my son-in-law. I rarely get to see Brad because his work keeps him in Los Angeles and my illness keeps me in Davis, but my gratitude runs deep. His wife may be an adult, but she's still my daughter and I think about her well-being all the time. Brad is such a loving and devoted husband and such a hard-working provider for his family that his presence in my life gives me one less thing to worry about, and this brings me peace of mind.

Malia—Mara and Brad's daughter. Malia was born five months before I got sick. She lights up my life even though I'm rarely able to see her. All I need once in a while is a "Hi, Nana" over the phone or an "I love you, Nana" in a text and my heart is full. I'm especially grateful to her for the good company she's been for Tony, her papa. They adore each other and when he's with her, his spirits are always lifted, giving him respite from his difficult role as caregiver for me.

Camden—Jamal and Bridgett's daughter. Oh, that special moment when I come out of the bedroom and see that Cam is visiting. She's growing up fast, but still brings young life, fresh life, into our house. She makes me glad to be alive.

Sylvia Boorstein—a founding teacher of Spirit Rock. Sylvia helped me learn to treat this illness with kindness and compassion. She also gave me invaluable support and help in moving the book from the manuscript stage to the publishing stage. My deepest gratitude to her is for the good friend she's been to Tony since I got sick. Those of you who have had the good fortune to know Sylvia will understand what I mean when I say that being in her "presence" (whether in person, by phone, or by email) is like being sprinkled with angel dust.

Kari Peterson—my good friend who possesses such a sharp and perceptive editor's eye. With the publication of this second edition, I've now been privileged to have Kari's invaluable feedback on the manuscripts for all three of my books.

Dawn Daro—my faithful friend. Our children grew up together, but then Dawn and I gradually grew apart. When she learned I was sick, she called me and we began to visit once a week, even if only for twenty minutes. Her steady presence in my life enriches it tremendously.

Richard Farrell—an undergrad with Tony and me at UC Riverside in the 1960s. After being out of touch with each other for over a decade, he moved back to Davis. It has rekindled the deepest of friendships. We can count on him. I hope he knows that he can count on us.

Jennie Spotila—my cyberspace friend whom I've never even talked to. Jennie is among the top patient advocates for ME/CFS. The work she does in that regard is vital to everyone with this bewildering illness. Jennie and I began casually emailing each other in 2015. Pretty soon we were exchanging emails almost every day. It has led to the deepest of friendships. We're here for each other, sharing our joys and sorrows in this life.

Dr. Paul Riggle—my primary care physician, who (as I like to tease him) drew the short straw when my doctor unexpectedly left while Tony and I were on that trip to Paris and I was randomly reassigned to him. Let me count the ways he is a gem: he listens, he never rushes me, he's open to new treatments, he's up to the challenge of having a patient he cannot "fix," he's compassionate. All this while having a huge patient load and a family of his own. He is the gold standard for doctors. He has never let me down. Never.

Doctors Richard Bold, Megan Daly, Helen Chew, and nurse practitioner Karen Natsuhara of the University of California–Davis Comprehensive Cancer Center. I could not be getting better care.

Dean Kevin Johnson and former dean Rex Perschbacher of UC Davis School of Law. Until my body just plain gave out, Rex and Kevin did everything they could to accommodate my illness, from allowing me to choose the best time of day to teach to replacing some classroom duties with administrative ones that I could perform from the bed. I'm grateful for their efforts and support.

Deon Vozov—who narrated all of my books, including both editions of this one. Deon reads my books the way I would if I had the talent and the skill. I know how unusual it is for the writer and the narrator to be a perfect match. But we are, and this is why I think of Deon as my sister.

Josh Bartok and Laura Cunningham—my editors at Wisdom Publications. I've been doubly blessed. Josh was the editor for the first edition of *How to Be Sick*, and Laura was the editor for this new edition. Both of them embody the qualities of a buddha—generosity, kindness, patience, wisdom, and equanimity.

Wisdom Publications—a special thank you to all the members of the Wisdom team for their wholehearted commitment to this book—especially Lydia Anderson, who worked so hard to promote Wisdom's impressive catalogue of offerings. I'm also grateful to Phil Pascuzzo for his exquisite cover designs for all of my books and to freelance editor Barry Boyce, who so beautifully polished the first edition of the book when the manuscript was in its final stages.

All my Dharma teachers—from those I've met in person to those I've studied under through their books. Thank you for the gift of the Buddha's teaching.

Recommended Reading

Aitken, Robert. *The Dragon Who Never Sleeps*
Aitken, Robert. *The Mind of Clover*
Batchelor, Martine. *The Spirit of the Buddha*
Batchelor, Stephen. *Buddhism Without Beliefs*
Beck, Charlotte Joko. *Everyday Zen*
Boorstein, Sylvia. *Happiness Is an Inside Job*
Boorstein, Sylvia. *It's Easier Than You Think*
Brach, Tara. *Radical Acceptance*
Buddhadasa, Bhikkhu. *Heartwood of the Bodhi Tree*
Chah, Ajahn. *Food for the Heart*
Chah, Ajahn. *A Still Forest Pool*
Chödrön, Pema. *Start Where You Are*
Chödrön, Pema. *The Wisdom of No Escape*
Dalai Lama, H. H. *Beyond Religion*
Goldstein, Joseph. *Insight Meditation*
Goldstein, Joseph, and Jack Kornfield. *Seeking the Heart of Wisdom*
Gunaratana, Bhante Henepola. *Mindfulness in Plain English*
Hanson, Rick. *Buddha's Brain*

Hart, William. *The Art of Living: Vipassana Meditation as Taught by S. N. Goenka*

Hass, Robert, editor. *The Essential Haiku: Versions of Basho, Buson, and Issa*

Kabat-Zinn, Jon. *Wherever You Go, There You Are*

Katie, Byron. *Loving What Is*

Khema, Ayya. *Being Nobody, Going Nowhere*

Khema, Ayya. *When the Iron Eagle Flies*

Macy, Joanna. *World as Lover, World as Self*

Miller, Karen Maezen. *Hand Wash Cold*

Mitchell, Stephen, editor. *The Enlightened Heart*

Nhat Hanh, Thich. *The Miracle of Mindfulness*

Nhat Hanh, Thich. *Present Moment Wonderful Moment*

Nhat Hanh, Thich. *The Sun My Heart*

Olendzki, Andrew. *Unlimiting Mind*

Olendzki, Andrew. *Untangling Self*

Rahula, Walpola. *What the Buddha Taught*

Richmond, Lewis. *Healing Lazarus*

Rumi, Maulana. *The Essential Rumi*. Translated by Coleman Barks with John Moyle

Ryokan. *Dewdrops on a Lotus Leaf*. Translated by John Stevens

Salzberg, Sharon. *Lovingkindness*

Seung, Sahn. *Dropping Ashes on the Buddha*

Sumedho, Ajahn. *The Mind and the Way*

Suzuki, Shunryu. *Zen Mind, Beginner's Mind*

Yamada, Koun. *The Gateless Gate*

Index

About the Author

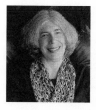

TONI BERNHARD is the author of *How to Live Well with Chronic Pain and Illness: A Mindful Guide* and *How to Wake Up: A Buddhist-Inspired Guide to Navigating Joy and Sorrow.* She's been interviewed on radio and for podcasts across the country and internationally. Her blog, "Turning Straw into Gold," is hosted by *Psychology Today* online. She maintains a personal relationship with her many thousands of fans on Facebook and other social media sites.

Toni fell ill on a trip to Paris in 2001 with what doctors initially diagnosed as an acute viral infection. She has not recovered. Until forced by illness to retire, she was a law professor at the University of California–Davis, serving six years as the dean of students.

She has been a practicing Buddhist since the early 1990s. She lives in Davis with her husband, Tony, and their gray Lab, Scout. Toni can be found online at www.tonibernhard.com.

What to Read Next
from Wisdom Publications

How to Live Well with Chronic Pain and Illness
A Mindful Guide
Toni Bernhard

"Toni shows us that difference between pain and suffering, and shows us what it can mean for how we live: that our lives can still be joyful."
—David R. Loy, author of *A New Buddhist Path*

How to Wake Up
A Buddhist-Inspired Guide to Navigating Joy and Sorrow
Toni Bernhard

"This is a book for everyone."
—Alida Brill, author of *Dancing at the River's Edge*

Relational Mindfulness
A Handbook for Deepening Our Connections with Ourselves, Each Other, and the Planet
Deborah Eden Tull

"A marvel of a book. Eden Tull meets us where we live: in constant interaction with self, other, world—and engagement with the challenges of a society in crisis."
—Joanna Macy, author of *Coming Back to Life*

Mindfulness in Plain English
20th Anniversary Edition
Bhante Gunaratana

"A masterpiece."
—Jon Kabat-Zinn

A Heart Full of Peace
Joseph Goldstein
Foreword by H. H. the Dalai Lama

"In this short but substantive volume, Joseph Goldstein, who lectures and leads retreats around the world, presents his thoughts on the practice of compassion, love, kindness, restraint, a skillful mind, and a peaceful heart as an antidote to the materialism of our age."
—*Spirituality & Practice*

Daily Wisdom
365 Buddhist Inspirations
Josh Bartok

"One of the basic practices of Buddhism is to remain mindful, and one way this is achieved is simply through reminders. Ranging in length from a sentence to a short page, these reminders include poetry, meditation instruction, practical advice, and thoughts on the way things are. Brilliant quotes from the likes of Ayya Khema, Alan Wallace, Milarepa, Henepola Gunaratana, Martine Batchelor, and the Dalai Lama. Retain this kind of inspiration throughout the day, and peace will be yours."
—Brian Bruya, religion editor, Amazon.com

Awake at the Bedside
Contemplative Teachings on Palliative and End-of-Life Care
Koshin Paley Ellison
Matt Weingast
Foreword by His Holiness the Karmapa, Ogyen Trinley Dorje

"The greatest degree of inner tranquility comes from the development of love and compassion. The more we care for the happiness of others, the greater is our own sense of well-being. Cultivating a close, warmhearted feeling for others automatically puts the mind at ease. It is the ultimate source of success in life. Awake at the Bedside supports this development of love and compassion."
—His Holiness the Dalai Lama

About Wisdom Publications

Wisdom Publications is the leading publisher of classic and contemporary Buddhist books and practical works on mindfulness. To learn more about us or to explore our other books, please visit our website at wisdompubs.org or contact us at the address below.

Wisdom Publications
199 Elm Street
Somerville, MA 02144 USA

We are a 501(c)(3) organization, and donations in support of our mission are tax deductible.

Wisdom Publications is affiliated with the Foundation for the Preservation of the Mahayana Tradition (FPMT).